"**M**ood disorders are so common few families escape having one or more members become victims. For them this book may be lifesaving. *The Mood Control Diet* is a modern prescription for diagnosing depression and for removing the major causes: malnutrition, special nutritional needs, food allergies, and chronic yeast infection. If you are depressed, you will save your health and your money by reading this book first. Do not leave home depressed, without it."

—ABRAM HOFFER, M.D., PH.D.,
president emeritus of the Huxley
Institute for Biosocial Research,
president of the Canadian
Schizophrenia Association, and editor-
in-chief of the *Journal of Orthomolecular
Medicine*

"**T**he authors skillfully translate a vast amount of contemporary scientific research into a practical, nutritional prescription that is certain to increase energy and alleviate negative mood states."

—PETER MILLER, PH.D., executive
director of The Hilton Head Health
Institute and author of *The Hilton Head
Metabolism Diet*

"**T**his book places a tool of great importance in the hands of people who recognize that what they eat must be wrong for them but cannot find the nutrition program that would make them healthy and happy again. Now they have the book that can show them how to eat their way out of their biochemical and nutritional problems."

—ALLAN COTT, M.D., author of *Dr. Cott's
Help for Your Learning-Disabled Child*

"*The Mood Control Diet* is a useful guide and extensive recipe book for those who want to help themselves to better health through proper diet."

—PRISCILLA A. SLAGLE, M.D.,
diplomate, American Board of
Psychiatry and Neurology

Also by Harvey M. Ross, M.D., and June Roth, M.S.:
The Executive Success Diet

Also by Harvey M. Ross, M.D.:
Hypoglycemia: The Disease Your Doctor Won't Treat
(coauthor, Jeraldine Saunders)

Fighting Depression

Also by June Roth, M.S.
Salt-free Cooking with Herbs and Spices
The Allergic Gourmet
Living Better with a Special Diet
Aerobic Nutrition (coauthor, Don Mannerberg, M.D.)
The Food/Depression Connection
The Pasta-Lover's Diet Book
Cooking for Your Hyperactive Child
Reversing Health Risks (coauthor, Julian Whitaker, M.D.)

THE

MOOD-CONTROL

DIET

21 Days to Conquering Depression and Fatigue

HARVEY M. ROSS, M.D.
AND
JUNE ROTH, M.S.

PRENTICE
HALL
PRESS

NEW YORK   LONDON   TORONTO
SYDNEY   TOKYO   SINGAPORE

PRENTICE HALL PRESS

15 Columbus Circle
New York, NY 10023

Copyright © 1990 by Harvey M. Ross, M.D., and June Roth, M.S.

PRENTICE HALL PRESS and colophons are registered trademarks
of Simon & Schuster, Inc.

Library of Congress Cataloging-in-Publication Data

Ross, Harvey M.
    The mood-control diet : 21 days to conquering
depression and fatigue / Harvey M. Ross and June Roth.—1st Prentice
Hall Press ed.
      p.   cm.
    Includes bibliographical references.
    ISBN 0-13-590449-8 (pbk.)
      1. Mental health—Nutritional aspects.   2. Depression, Mental—
Diet therapy.   3. Fatigue—Diet therapy.   I. Roth, June
II. Title.   III. Title: Mood-control diet.
RC455.4.N8R67   1990
616.85'270654—dc20   89-25540
                                          CIP

Designed by Robert Bull Design

Manufactured in the United States of America

10 9 8 7 6 5 4 3 2 1

First Paperback Edition

In memory of Jan Michael "Derek" Kennedy

CONTENTS

WHAT THIS BOOK WILL DO FOR YOU

Dear Reader,

The relationship between food sensitivities and mental and physical health has fascinated me for many years. During that time, I researched and wrote several books that linked food with behavioral reactions. Reader mail in response to my syndicated newspaper column "Special Diets/Nutrition Hotline" is always particularly heavy whenever I write about a facet of this theory.

When discussing the problems of chronic depression and fatigue with Harvey M. Ross, M.D., a psychiatrist who specializes in treatment that takes into account his patients' nutritional histories, we decided to coauthor this book. We are each imbued with the desire to teach people how to understand their own biochemical uniqueness and find the nutrition program that makes them feel and be their best.

There are several mood and energy disorders directly related to diet. Many people don't even know they are suffering from one of these problems, but often it is an underlying cause of chronic fatigue, mood swings, and depression. Our three-step Mood-Control Diet addresses these disorders in detail, while letting you enjoy a wide variety of foods. The recipe section is devised to give you delicious meals designed specifically to combat food-related illnesses. It will keep your menus interesting as you change your way of eating to improve your health. As a clinical nutritionist, I am confident that you will be well nourished as you detoxify from foods that may be contributing to feelings of lethargy and lack of verve.

The Mood-Control Diet is also excellent for those people who know that they have a poor diet but don't know how to improve it. This book provides an easy-to-follow step-by-step dietary program that is presented in a detailed practical manner. The Mood-Control Diet allows you to gradually improve your diet to the benefit of your physical and mental well-being.

It is my hope that this book will help you to detect and resolve nutrition-related problems so you can control your moods and health forevermore, finding new levels of energy and vitality.

Warmly,
June Roth, M.S.
Teaneck, New Jersey

FOREWORD

This book is for you if you or anyone close to you have ever been depressed and the usual treatments failed to offer significant relief or if you have ever been fatigued to a point where your enjoyment of life was compromised and repeated medical examinations and laboratory tests indicated that you should be feeling great.

I believe that the program provided in this book can help bring happiness and energy back into your life.

For more than twenty years I have been working with people who have experienced depression and fatigue and have not responded to the usual treatments of psychotherapy and antidepressant medications. Early in my career in psychiatry, I questioned the prevailing thinking that if you were depressed, something (perhaps hidden causes in one's background) caused that depression. I was not alone in my doubts about the psyche being the exclusive source of depression. By sharing findings and experiences with my colleagues and by listening to my patients, I was able to discover hidden causes for some depressions and fatigue that remain prevalent in our society and that are strongly connected to our daily diets.

The solutions found in the following pages are neither the end nor the beginning of our research, but somewhere in between. As time passes more will be learned, techniques will be perfected for easier and more exacting diagnosis, and treatments will be fine-tuned. What follows is what we know today of some of the most common and most overlooked causes of depression and fatigue.

I have had the great satisfaction, when applying the principles outlined in these chapters, of seeing people who were at the point of despair, return to happy, energetic, and productive lives. I feel privileged to share this information with you.

Harvey M. Ross, M.D.
Los Angeles, California

THE
MOOD-CONTROL
DIET

PART ONE

INTRODUCING THE PROGRAM

1

WHEN THE DOCTOR SAYS YOU'RE OKAY
DESPITE THE BLAHS

T HOUSANDS OF PEOPLE SUFFER FROM chronic depression and fatigue, searching desperately for the reason behind their problems. Often they are told there is nothing wrong with them and that the problem must have a psychological, not a medical, cause. Yet for many, therapy doesn't work. It doesn't work because it doesn't address the real cause of certain chronic malaises, which lies in the biochemical/nutritional framework. Only a lucky few find a physician with a background that includes an awareness that medical/nutritional factors often play an important part in causing depression and fatigue.

A doctor who is tuned in to the link between a patient's unexplained problems and yeast infections, food sensitivities, hypoglycemia, and nutritional deprivation can do a world of good when treating depression and fatigue. This book is designed to reveal how these disorders may be nutritionally based and what you can do about it.

"DON'T WORRY, EVERYTHING IS ALL RIGHT"—THE STORY OF FRAN

After her doctor told her, "All the tests are normal. Everything is all right," Fran was on the verge of tears. Not from happiness and relief, but from the frustration of not getting any answers—answers she knew were there somewhere. For the past few years, Fran had known she was not all right. She felt much older than her thirty-five years, she had had to give up her secretarial job, and her marriage was definitely in jeopardy. Her moodiness and feelings of fatigue resulted in lack of sexual interest most of the time. She *knew* she was *not* "all right."

Fran's problems became noticeable after delivering her second child. She was unable to concentrate, felt blue more often than she should, and got upset over the smallest frustrations. Worst of all, her energy was almost nonexistent. She could take care of her baby, but was unable to perform any

3

other household work. After a few months she did consult her physician who told her she was suffering from postpartum depression and that it would go away as quickly as it came. It didn't. Although her plan had always been to return to work after several months at home with her baby, she was unable even to consider the possibility.

When the depression didn't lift as she was told it would; when her energy level became worse and her mood bleaker, she consulted another physician. A complete physical and routine blood work was done, and she heard for the first time the litany that was to be repeated by her physicians and consultants over the next few years—"All the tests are normal."

After a few years of normal tests and no significant reduction in her fatigue and depression, Fran was advised by her physician to consult a psychiatrist. The reasoning was that nothing of an abnormal nature could be found in her blood tests and yet she was obviously suffering from something. The problem must be a mental or emotional illness, which was in the province of psychiatry.

The psychiatrist was sympathetic, knowledgeable—and ineffective. After a few sessions of history taking and some psychological testing, the psychiatrist, a motherly woman in her mid-fifties, suggested a course of psychotherapy and antidepressant medication. For the first few weeks, Fran felt relieved, happy, and thankful that she was finally in good hands. Help was being given, and she was hopeful that there was some light at the end of a tunnel that had been completely black for so long.

Fran's hopes were short lived. The medication made her drowsy, and even though she was encouraged to continue taking it with the promise that the drowsiness would abate, she remained lethargic and later developed tremors. A series of medication changes occurred over the next several months. Fran did experience some elevation of her mood, but she also had side effects—drowsiness, confusion, dry mouth, constipation, weight gain, and headaches—which made it impossible to continue with the medication. She knew antidepressants were effective for some people, but not for her. Psychotherapy was discontinued by mutual consent when she and her doctor both agreed everything had been tried and no progress was being made.

Fran was reluctant to leave the care of the doctor whom she liked so much, but she knew something else had to be done. A friend of Fran's had been a patient of Dr. Ross. She suggested that Fran make an appointment, because so many of the complaints that Fran expressed were the same ones the friend had had before seeing Dr. Ross. At the time of the first interview, Fran recited her familiar complaints of depression, fatigue, and mental confusion involving memory, concentration, and decision-making abilities. She was surprised at some of the questions posed by Dr. Ross. They seemed out of place and even somewhat irrelevant. For example, Dr. Ross asked her whether there was a presence or frequency of yeast infections, whether her periods were regular and how heavy they were, whether she had ever used antibiotics and birth control pills, and how her symptoms changed prior to her period and during her pregnancy. After taking a thorough physical and nutritional history, Dr. Ross told her that he suspected a sensitivity to yeast. He ordered a blood test to confirm her body's immune system's response to yeast. When the test revealed a positive immune response to yeast, Dr. Ross began appropriate antiyeast treatment (explained in detail in chapters 5 and 10). Within three weeks, Fran began to feel better. Her depression lifted significantly, energy returned, and she recognized her "old self" again. The therapeutic program with some modifications was continued for about three years. Most of that time Fran felt well. She returned to work, still had plenty of energy to spend with her children, and her marriage regained its vitality.

Fran's illness, and the havoc brought on her family as well as herself, is fairly typical. Her frustration at being told, "All the tests are normal," is a scenario repeated daily in physicians' offices all over the country. Psychiatrists' offices are filled with the results of other physicians' frustrations—those patients who just don't feel well, don't respond to treatment, and yet in whom no abnormalities can be found on the examining table or in the laboratory. Psychiatry for this group of patients usually results in frustration for the psychiatrists and for the patients, who often feel that psychiatric treatment is the last and final hope. Fortunately, there is more: There is hope, and there is a better approach.

"MY BOSS AND FRIENDS MUST THINK I'M CRAZY!"—THE STORY OF ROBERT

A better approach was also found by Robert, a thirty-six-year-old, hard-working single man who was referred to Dr. Ross by his psychologist, who believed all of Robert's problems could not be psychological. Robert had started psychotherapy for a depression that he had been battling for two to three years. He was unable to pinpoint when it started, but recognized that he had been slowing down over that time period. He had gradually withdrawn from social contacts and kept to himself more and more while working in a large accounting firm. He fought hard to control bouts of irritability that he didn't understand. He had always been a friendly individual, popular, and easy to get along with. He suffered headaches for about a year, sometimes relieved by simple pain killers, sometimes not. A physical examination and special neurologic examinations found nothing physical to explain the headaches. Robert tried to learn to live with them, but he found that to be impossible.

His physician suggested psychotherapy because no physical explanations were found. By the time Robert sought help from the psychologist, he was functioning at a very poor level. At work, he felt more fake than functional, and he learned how to get through the day without drawing too much attention to himself. He became anxious, feeling it was just a matter of time before his poor performance would be noticed. He knew he couldn't get by on his previously good work performance forever.

The psychologist who heard Robert's history felt there was no catastrophic life event significant enough to account for the level of dysfunction Robert was experiencing. Certainly he had some worries about his job and relationships, but those worries came after the problems started, not before. After two months of weekly psychotherapy, the psychologist concluded that Robert was open and aware and that there were no past dark secrets or buried problems of any degree that resulted in Robert's dysfunctioning.

Because all the physical laboratory examinations had always been normal and the psychologist felt the problem was not psychological in origin, he suggested Robert consult Dr. Ross, who had experience in treating problems using a nutritional approach. (The psychologist was alerted to this avenue of treatment by his own problems that had been helped significantly a number of years before by such an approach.)

When Dr. Ross heard Robert's dietary habits, the diagnosis became clear. He found that Robert ate irregularly, rarely eating breakfast and often skipping lunch. He did eat snacks frequently, but only when he felt weak during the day. The snacks were usually soft drinks, candy, or anything else that would not only satisfy Robert's sweet tooth, but would also relieve his weakness and mental fuzziness. Dr. Ross became suspicious that Robert had hypoglycemia (low blood sugar), a condition in which the body's ability to stabilize blood sugar levels no longer works. The effect is that the body's blood sugar falls to a very low level, resulting in all the physical and mental symptoms Robert was experiencing. Dr. Ross confirmed this diagnosis using a five-hour glucose tolerance test.

Within three months after following the Mood-Control Diet, outlined in chapter 10, Robert felt as well as he had ever felt. As long as he is sensible with his diet, knowing when to be strict and when he might be a little lax, he stays well and has no problems.

If you suspect that you might have hypoglycemia, you will find an in-depth discussion of this disease in chapter 3, "Get Off the Glucose Roller Coaster."

"I'M SO TIRED I COULD DIE"— THE STORY OF LORI

Lori, a well-dressed, attractive woman in her early thirties, held a high-powered job as the business manager of a large and busy law firm, a position she had had for about four years. Until the previous year, she had enjoyed her work, which was physically and emotionally demanding. At first, she noticed she was getting tired more frequently and the amount of sleep she got did not seem to help. Some months later, she felt depressed and began to complain about the workload and withdraw from social contacts. Her bosses suggested a month's vacation. Lori did feel well while on vacation, but within a week of returning it was as if she had never gone away. She was alarmed by other symptoms that appeared: some swelling and aching of her finger joints and a skin rash on her torso. A visit to her physician did not provide any real answer. Her laboratory tests were normal, her physical examination was unchanged from two years previously, with the exception of the rash, and a fifteen-pound weight gain. The weight gain bothered her, but after trying a low-calorie diet for a few weeks and losing only two pounds, Lori felt she didn't have the energy to continue with a program that resulted in such a paltry weight loss. Her physician ordered a mild tranquilizer to curb her anxiety and a cortisone cream for her rash. The tranquilizer made her sleepy and made it more difficult for her to function. The cortisone cream seemed to be of very limited help, so she stopped using it. It was at this point that Lori was referred to Dr. Ross.

Dr. Ross asked Lori to outline her eating patterns in detail. Because she had not been feeling well, she had not been paying much attention to her diet. She had no interest in food and no energy to prepare food for herself. Whenever she was hungry she drank a glass of milk. She also ate crackers and cold cereal with milk, no sugar. She ate bread and butter twice a day. About five times a week she did manage to eat a frozen dinner at home. Once a week, she might dine out with friends, selecting fish or chicken and a salad.

Lori's history revealed a long period during her childhood when she experienced allergies. As an infant, she had a milk allergy, but seemed to grow out of it later in her childhood. Her family, including two of her four siblings, her mother, and several members of the maternal side of her family, were prone to both food and airborne allergies.

Dr. Ross ordered appropriate testing to determine whether Lori was suffering from food sensitivities. He suspected these because of Lori's emotional system, joint aches, and skin rash, accompanied by her previous history of allergies and a strong family disposition for allergies. The tests showed a significant allergic response to wheat, milk, halibut (the fish Lori always ordered when dining out), broccoli, tomatoes, and cheddar cheese.

Lori was started on the Mood-Control Diet, eliminating the foods to which she was found to be sensitive. At first she found the diet very difficult and craved milk and bread, but she found feeling bad even more difficult and so she stayed with the program. Within only a week, she began to notice some encouraging changes that motivated her to continue. She lost five pounds and was delighted, because in the past year she had not been able to lose weight without lowering her calories to less than 800 calories a day. She also noted that she was not at all hungry on this program. By the end of three weeks, Lori was beginning to feel normal again. She estimated that her rash and fatigue symptoms were about 90 percent gone. The offending foods were slowly reintroduced after about four months. She became aware of the food-mood connection and learned that as long as she didn't consume milk and bread more than once every four days, she remained symptom-free.

There are many more cases like Fran's, Robert's, and Lori's, most with a happy outcome. Many times, people who have suffered with depression and fatigue, often over long periods of time, and who have been told that "the tests are normal" are victims of not having the correct tests done. These tests are discussed in chapter 4, "Why Good Food May Be Bad for You."

Patients are discouraged and lose hope when they hear they are "normal" as a result of routine medical testing. If the suspicion is high for a medical-nutritional cause for fatigue and depression and the correct tests are done, the doctor will be able to say, "I'm happy to tell you, your tests are 'abnormal' and there is a good chance we can do something about it!"

The following chapter offers a series of self-assessment tests that will provide the first clue in the detective work needed to assess your own food-mood history.

2

FIVE QUICK STEPS TO PINPOINT
YOUR MOOD PROBLEMS

Depression and fatigue are not always caused by the same problem. They can spring from medical, psychological, or food-related sources and sometimes they result from a combination of several disorders. That's why patients often end up going from doctor to doctor, trying to get to the cause so they can do something to regain their energy and vitality.

Some years ago, depression was thought to have a psychological cause. Today, with the exception of a few remaining hotbeds of strict psychoanalytic thinking, the consensus is that depression may result from a multitude of causes ranging from the purely medical, purely food related or nutritional, or purely psychological. The diagnosis becomes more difficult when depression and fatigue come from multiple causes.

The successful treatment of depression and the restoration of full energy depends on a careful determination of the basic causes of the depression. The treatment must fit the cause, not the theoretical orientation of the health professional.

Too often, the preliminary work of finding the cause of depression and fatigue falls on the shoulders of the person experiencing the problems. While it is important to participate in your own diagnosis, it is unfair when the therapist's rigid treatment orientation blocks out the investigation of every possible diagnostic avenue.

Carefully consider your symptoms and answer the questions in this chapter to raise or lower suspicions for some of the most overlooked causes of depression and fatigue. When you uncover some clues, you will be better able to get some help or help yourself.

STEP 1: IS IT PSYCHOLOGICAL OR MEDICAL?

For a person who is depressed, the first question that differentiates medical from psychological causes is:

_____ Is there anything that has happened in your life that easily accounts for the degree of depression you are experiencing?

In depressions resulting from psychological causes, there is usually a clear life event that accounts not only for the depression, but also for the degree of the depression. Many times, in an attempt to assign a cause to a troubling depression, people will focus on some unpleasantness in their lives, but they have a gut feeling, "I shouldn't be this depressed about that." They are usually correct. The purely psychological cause for depression is usually easily identified by a major loss or change.

Ask yourself these questions:

_____ Have you recently lost a mate?

_____ Have you recently lost a close relative or friend?

_____ Are you having difficulties in a relationship?

_____ Are you experiencing a loss of self-esteem?

_____ Have you recently changed jobs?

_____ Are you deeply unhappy about your working conditions?

_____ Have you had financial reverses?

_____ Have you moved your residence to another city and are finding it difficult to readjust your life?

While the focus of this book is on eradicating food-related problems, it's important to find out whether the cause of your particular problem is what you're eating, or what's eating you! If a suspected life problem exists but does not easily explain the degree of depression you are experiencing, then look for a medical or nutritional cause.

To rule out a medical cause, have your doctor conduct a complete medical examination. Find out whether you have abnormal (high or low) blood sugar, low thyroid, what your blood pressure is, whether your cholesterol is at or below the desired 200-mg level, whether you have high blood triglycerides, and whether there is any other irregularity showing up in your blood and urine samples. Also ask your doctor to determine whether you are overweight or underweight and in shape or out of shape, based on the norms for your age, sex, and activity level.

If it is not a psychological or medical problem, you may be suffering from one, or several, of four common—but often overlooked—causes for depression. By answering the questions that follow in steps 2 through 5, you can get a head start on tracking down the possible cause of your depression and/or fatigue.

STEP 2: IS IT A HYPOGLYCEMIA-RELATED FOOD DISORDER?

One of the most common food-related causes of depression is hypoglycemia—low blood sugar. In chapter 3, you will find out how to get control of hypoglycemia if it has control over you. Suspect hypoglycemia if you answer yes to several of the following questions.

____ Do you have a definite sweet tooth?

____ Do you overindulge in alcohol?

____ Do you crave starchy food?

____ Is there a history in your family of alcoholism, diabetes, or hypo-glycemia?

____ Does sugar pick you up when you are feeling very weak?

____ Does sugar pick you up when you have trouble concentrating and making decisions?

STEP 3: IS IT A FOOD-SENSITIVITY-RELATED DISORDER?

Another food-related cause of depression and fatigue can be food sensitivities. In chapter 4, you will learn several methods of detecting a trigger food (the food substance to which you are sensitive), including the 4-Day Food-Rotation Plan whereby no food or its related food family members are eaten more than once every four days. Suspect food sensitivities if you answer yes to several of the following questions.

____ Do you have a strong history of allergies?

____ Do you come from a very allergic family?

____ Are there a number of foods which you eat several times a week, or even several times daily?

____ Do you have physical problems, such as skin, respiratory, digestive, or bone and joint problems that have not been helped significantly by medical attention?

Do you have trouble losing weight, even when you stay on a low-calorie diet?

STEP 4: IS IT A YEAST-INFECTION-RELATED DISORDER?

It is amazing to find how many cases of depression and fatigue are caused by yeast infections. In chapter 5, you will learn how to eat defensively when plagued with side effects of yeast and fungus foods. These are foods that depend on fermenting or bacterial action, such as yeast breads and cakes, Roquefort cheese, and mushrooms. You can suspect possible yeast reactions if you answer yes to several of the following questions.

For women:

_____ Have you had numerous yeast infections?

_____ Are your menstrual periods irregular?

_____ Is the flow during your period either heavy or lighter than it should be?

_____ Are you now, or have you been, on birth control pills?

_____ Are you taking progesterone?

_____ Do you experience frequent urinary tract infections?

For men and women:

_____ Do you have abdominal bloating after eating?

_____ Do you experience some diarrhea and some constipation?

_____ Are you particularly sensitive to strong perfumes and to smog, causing breathing difficulties?

_____ Do you have frequent hoarseness problems?

_____ Have you taken a lot of antibiotics?

STEP 5: IS IT A POOR-NUTRITION-RELATED DISORDER?

It is possible that your only problem is that you have poor eating habits and may be in a state of subnutrition. The human body can't function without necessary nutrients (this situation is discussed in chapter 6). You can stop paying that piper forever using this book. You may be shortchanging your body of needed nutrients if you eat a lot of processed foods, frozen dinners, habitually eat on the run in fast-food restaurants, or frequently follow too-stringent low-calorie diets. Suspect a condition of general subnutrition if you can answer yes to several of the following questions.

___ Do you eat a lot of junk food?

___ Do you eat a bare minimum because of appetite or dieting to lose weight?

___ Do you only eat a few foods, disliking a variety of foods?

___ Do you rarely eat fresh vegetables?

___ Do you rarely eat fresh fruits?

___ Do you rarely eat whole grains?

___ Do you have several alcoholic drinks a week?

___ Do you smoke tobacco?

___ Do you avoid taking nutritional supplements?

These five quick steps can help you pinpoint what is causing your mood problems. By carefully considering the questions, you can take advantage of the clues they reveal. You should be able to suspect whether the depression and fatigue you experience are caused by psychological, medical, and/or nutritional reasons.

Besides these four commonly overlooked causes of depression, there are other medical causes, such as Epstein-Barr Syndrome, thyroid dysfunction, and other physically debilitating diseases as well as genetic predisposition, that result in significant depressive states. Chapter 20 (Special Problem and Food-Fixer Section) includes information to alert you to other food-related possibilities. Because a complete discussion of these disorders lies outside the scope of this book, we recommend getting a thorough medical workup to rule them out.

Now that you have pinpointed the food-related causes of your depression or fatigue, let's explore how the body's nutrient delivery system works so you can provide your body's unique nutritional needs and banish the blahs forever!

3

GET OFF THE GLUCOSE ROLLER COASTER

HYPOGLYCEMIA (LOW BLOOD SUGAR) HAS been in and out of favor as a diagnosis since it was first recognized in the 1920s by Dr. Seale Harris. Initially Dr. Harris was commended for his discovery of this condition. In the 1950s, the heyday of psychosomatic diagnosis, physicians attributed many physical and emotional complaints to hypoglycemia. Later, when the practice of medicine became drug oriented, the hypoglycemia diagnosis became unpopular.

By the late 1960s and 1970s, the emerging interest in nutrition and its effect on health and disease caused the "rediscovery" of hypoglycemia, particularly by the public. In fact, doctors were so bombarded by patients who had read about this illness in magazines and books they dubbed hypoglycemia a "fad disease."

The arguments still continue over whether to categorize hypoglycemia as the "scourge to mankind" or to relegate it to the "no disease" category. The truth, as many truths, lies somewhere in between. It is true that some people went overboard in attributing all their problems to hypoglycemia. But labeling a known condition as a fad does not eliminate its existence any more than not believing in war or poverty can eliminate those problems. Although at one time the condition might have been overdiagnosed, it is a valid diagnosis for many people.

If your doctor answers your questions about hypoglycemia with any of the popular hypoglycemic myths listed below, it's time to get a second opinion. Caveat emptor!

HYPOGLYCEMIA MYTHS

- Hypoglycemia does not exist/is very rare.
- All you have to do to treat hypoglycemia is stop eating sugar.
- The treatment for hypoglycemia is to suck on candy when you feel weak.
- You should have a little more sugar in your diet to keep your blood sugar up.

Hypoglycemia is the result of the failure of the stabilizing mechanisms of the body to maintain a proper blood sugar (glucose) level after a person has eaten. Hypoglycemic symptoms occur either when the blood sugar drops to a point that is too low for maintaining proper nourishment of the nervous and muscular systems or when the blood sugar level drops too rapidly. The symptoms of hypoglycemia may be divided into immediate and long-term categories. The immediate group consists of a pronounced, profound weakness, sometimes a rubbery-leg feeling, and/or some confusion and inability to think clearly. Decision making is cumbersome, if possible at all. These symptoms occur when the blood sugar reaches a low level. They are blissfully relieved as suddenly as they occur by a simple maneuver: eating. Most of us experience these symptoms if we wait too long to eat. In most cases, although symptoms are annoying, they are not serious or long lasting.

It is the symptoms that fall into the long-term group that can wreak havoc in daily life and send a person on a medical odyssey, visiting one physician after the other looking for relief. The symptoms in this group usually do not occur rapidly and require much more than just one good meal to overcome them. A study of 500 people with hypoglycemia demonstrated that fully 99 percent of them complained of fatigue; about 75 percent were depressed; an equal percentage complained of anxiety attacks; and more than 50 percent had some type of bodily pain, which ranged from headaches, extremity pains, chest pains often mimicking heart attacks, and abdominal pains often mistakenly diagnosed as ulcers. A very small percentage of those questioned had experienced fainting and convulsions. Irritability was present in a high percentage of those diagnosed with hypoglycemia.

These long-range symptoms occur only when the blood sugar level has fallen repeatedly over a long period of time. They are not produced rapidly and it takes some time to overcome them. In most cases, however, after three twenty-one-day periods of proper treatment, complete health can be restored.

Most of the time, hypoglycemia is the result of a large intake of refined carbohydrates, such as sugar, alcohol, and enriched white flour, over the course of many months or years by someone who is genetically predisposed to having the disorder. Most of us greatly underestimate the amount of sugar we eat. Many people think that if they don't add sugar to their coffee, they aren't eating any sugar worth mentioning.

If you read the labels on packaged food products, however, you will be amazed by how many synonyms manufacturers can come up with for sugar: Sucrose, dextrose, natural sweeteners, and syrups are just a few examples. It is not unusual to find three out of the first five ingredients listed on a label (in order of the relative amount of that item in the product) are refined carbohydrates. Sugar is a part of so many packaged foods that the smallest source of your sugar intake is from the sugar bowl! Being aware of the hidden sources of sugar in your diet is a big step toward bringing hypoglycemia under control. Our program will alert you to the hidden sugars in your diet, so you can beat the sugar blues at their own game.

TREATING HYPOGLYCEMIA

If you know what you are doing, the treatment for hypoglycemia is fairly simple. Our Mood-Control Diet with the hypoglycemia modification of frequent snacks, plus the addition of a high potency multivitamin and mineral supplement containing chromium, is the only program necessary to change a suffering hypoglycemic into an energetic, happy person.

Sometimes it is easier said than done. You can't expect to eat one meal or even several days of meals and feel like a new person. Patience and persistence do pay off, but each person has a unique chemistry and some hypoglycemics go through several mood stages before their blood sugar stops yo-yoing. Therefore it is important to overcome the natural tendency to expect immediate gratification and accept a more realistic scenario. It will be worth the effort.

WHAT TO EXPECT USING THE MOOD-CONTROL DIET

After a few healthy meals, many hypoglycemics expect to feel like a new person. It doesn't happen that way. By overcoming the natural tendency to expect immediate gratification and accepting a more realistic scenario, it is easier to be both patient and persistent. Your body needs time to readjust. Be patient with yourself!

Dr. Ross has created three twenty-one-day segments in his course of treatment. Each segment has its own characteristics. Once you understand what to expect during each of these segments, you can be guided more by reality than by false expectations. Close associates and family members also can be supportive when they know what to expect.

THE FIRST STAGE

The first stage is perversely the most difficult. Most people, instead of feeling better, feel worse. They experience an increase of hypoglycemia's two main symptoms: fatigue and depression. Most people in stage 1 can expect to feel worse at first, resulting in less energy and more depression. Expecting this to happen has helped people tolerate the program, and has helped family and friends accept a worsening of the depression and fatigue initially. Don't be frightened off by knowing things will get worse before they get better. Feeling worse in this case is part of the process of feeling better. Only 5 percent of people have a profound loss of energy; most others realize that although they feel worse, there is no significant interference with their activities, which often weren't so great before the program.

There seems to be a direct correlation with the amount of sugar people consume before starting the program and their experience of depression and fatigue in this first stage. The more sugar you had been consuming the worse you may initially feel on this program. Remember, most people consume much more sugar than they realize.

Something else you may encounter during the first stage is a strong sugar craving. It is important to know that this craving is not going to be lifelong! By following the Mood-Control Diet, the craving for sugar lasts only three weeks, although it might reoccur briefly when your day-to-day stress level increases. If this happens to you, ride it through—the situation will get better!

THE SECOND STAGE

Once you have accomplished the first twenty-one-day segment, week 3 of the Mood-Control Diet becomes your maintenance program. As to your mood, the second twenty-one-day-segment starts very abruptly. You may awaken one morning and everything seems great. The depression has lifted and your energy level is anywhere from good to bordering on the hyperactive. Much to your dismay, however, by midafternoon the bottom seems to drop out and you may feel a sudden loss of energy and a surge of depression. This cycle is repeated after a few days and again in another few days. Throughout, keep in mind that this is normal for stage 2. Keep following week 3 of the Mood-Control Diet to the letter. Provided you are undergoing no other inordinate physical or emotional stresses, the ups and downs will start to flatten out. By the end of this twenty-one-day period, rapid fluctuations in your mood and energy levels are no longer taking place. Although your mood now is good, you may find that your energy is still low. Some people, not expecting this opposing movement of mood and energy, feel discouraged and question the entire program, noting that they felt more energetic during the beginning of the second stage.

How to keep going? Remember that the second twenty-one-day period is characterized by rapid changes in mood and energy. The timing of the changes may vary from once every few days lasting for several hours (which is the most common pattern) to changes occurring every several days, lasting for several days. The length or frequency of the changes is not significant; the fact that changes are occurring is an important indication that treatment is progressing successfully.

Two important hints have helped many people at the second stage. The first is to live one day at a time—or better, one hour at a time! Because the changes are so rapid, you cannot predict your mood or energy level one hour in advance or sometimes even ten minutes in advance. So don't fill your calendar with a dozen appointments and plans as soon as you feel well. You don't want to be caught up in obligations that you don't have the energy or interest to fulfill. Enjoy the up mood when it occurs and accept the depression and fatigue when they return. They will not be your constant companions; don't let them throw you!

The second hint is don't overreact to the changes. It is tempting to think that everything has been cured when you wake up feeling exceptionally well. Conversely, when the low feelings suddenly return, a feeling of discouragement can complicate your treatment by adding a burden of psychological stress.

THE THIRD STAGE

After the ups and downs of the second stage, one slips quietly into the third twenty-one-day segment, still following the week-3 menu plan. This is the pay-off stage! It is characterized by subtle, but stable and gradual, improvement in energy. There are no great ups here, but rather a steady increase in energy, which is often noted after the fact. You may notice tasks that have gone undone for lack of energy are now done without a second thought. Closets and drawers get cleaned, yards get put back into shape, telephone calls are returned without your having to be "psyched up" to do it. You find that you no longer have to ration your energy. You are moving forward in life, rather than riding the brake.

If you continue to follow the Mood-Control Diet your symptoms of hypoglycemia will remain under control. A good mood and sufficient energy will be the rule rather than the exception.

NO MORE SUGAR FOREVER?

Let's be realistic. Very few of us mortals can start a diet and stay with it forever. Sometimes we go off the diet by design, sometimes we do it inadvertently. But going off the diet need not mean that you are going to feel lousy. If you do it wisely, you can depart from the program without significant negative effects.

The secret? The effect of dietary lapses depends much more on frequency than it does on the amount of food eaten. A small amount of refined carbohydrates eaten every few days will not cause symptoms of fatigue and depression. Doing this, however, will not improve your energy levels.

A better solution is to have one free day a week and to follow the Mood-Control Diet carefully for the other six. On the seventh day, you may eat any food in any amount without compromising the program's overall positive results.

When you allow for a free day, two things happen. First, many people get a boost from taking a break. No longer is it necessary to say, "I can never have a piece of pie à la mode. I can never have a soft drink." These people find it is easier to follow the program for six days when they can look forward to a special treat on the seventh day.

Second, a free day can teach you volumes about the deleterious effect of sugar. During the first two weeks on the diet, you will not usually have any noticeable physical effects from your free day. From about the third week on, however, if you consume refined carbohydrates or alcohol on your free day, you will feel a reaction. You will have a feeling of fatigue, some depression, and perhaps some irritability. This reaction lasts twenty-four hours and usually starts the day after eating the refined carbohydrates. About 10 to 15 percent of the time the reaction starts forty-eight to seventy-two hours later. The reaction always lasts one day, but it never reverses the overall beneficial effects of the program.

You may look forward to your free days, but many people after two or three such experiences say, "It's not worth it." They discover that the Mood-Control Diet doesn't take foods away from them so much as it gives them something valuable: the good feeling of feeling good. At that point, staying with the Mood-Control Diet and collecting the rewards becomes easy.

For a few people, returning to the program after their free day is onerous. For this small group of people, the one-day diet vacation is not a good idea. People who fall into this group usually know who they are and realize that the free-day plan is not good for them.

By following the Mood-Control Diet, you can eradicate the depression and fatigue caused by hypoglycemia. Your busy life can be resumed in a spirit of confidence with a clear head, a good mood, and sufficient energy to accomplish whatever has to be done.

Stay with the third week's menu plan ever after. It will stabilize your blood glucose level. The third week menu plan is your maintenance program. Be assured, there is calm and peace at the end of this special-diet rainbow!

4

WHY GOOD FOOD MAY BE BAD FOR YOU

"I ONLY EAT GOOD FOODS. I NEVER TOUCH junk, and it has been more than three years since I've had a drink." Being a model of nutritional propriety, George couldn't understand why he had daily headaches, abdominal discomfort, depression, and a persistent tiredness that he overcame by enormous willpower during the day at his office but which caused him to spend most evenings and weekends "resting" in bed. Decisions, even minor ones, at his law office were presenting major problems, and he found himself discouraging prospective new clients. At home, his failure to participate in family activities, lack of sexual interest, and inability to contribute to the day-to-day functioning of the household had estranged him from his children and wife. There had even been some discussion of a separation.

George's wife, Mary, having watched his deterioration over a three-year period, believed that he must be having a medical problem. At her insistence, and because he was too tired to refuse, George finally allowed Mary to contact his physician. His doctor performed a complete physical and ordered the routine blood tests, which had not been done for about four years.

Both George and Mary had mixed feelings about the physician's conclusion: "I can't find anything wrong with you. You have absolutely normal tests. You've got the blood pressure of a twenty year old." They were relieved that no serious illness was found, but the doctor's examination hadn't explained why George felt so ill. A neurologist was consulted about George's persistent headaches, but that examination was also pronounced normal. George felt he was the sickest "normal" man he had ever known!

Mary brought George to Dr. Ross's office on the advice of a good friend who had been a patient of Dr. Ross. George was a reluctant client. He didn't want to be told again, "There's nothing wrong." He knew something wasn't right, but he was losing faith that anyone would be able to confirm his suspicions.

During the first interview, several important pieces of George's history were uncovered. George came from a very allergic family. Both maternal and paternal sides were filled with relatives who suffered from ordinary seasonal allergies as well as food allergies. George had been an allergic infant and had had trouble throughout his childhood, but he seemed to outgrow these problems in his early teens and adulthood.

George had experienced various minor aches and pains, but had never paid much attention to them because they were not disabling, and George was not a complainer. When questioned, he mentioned that he had gained about fifteen pounds over the last five years and had had a terrible time trying to shed those pounds, even with a low-calorie diet and increased exercise. The weight, which had never been a problem earlier in his life, was disturbing. George had always been proud of his physique and the extra weight was not in keeping with his self-image. When diet and exercise failed to produce the results he wanted, his wife suggested that they both go to a spa. During the two-week period, Mary cheated and still lost eight pounds. George obeyed the diet to the letter, but lost only three pounds. Even that loss was short-lived: Within ten days of his return home, he had gained five pounds. At that point he gave up any further efforts at weight loss, but was not happy about it.

A review of George's eating habits, which he considered good, was interesting. It was true that he didn't eat any of the major dietary offenders: caffeine, alcohol, sugar, and enriched white flour. Nor did he use tobacco. George was not very interested in food; he chose what he considered to be good food, but he never varied his selections. Every morning he ate hot whole-grain oatmeal. He had at least three pieces of whole-grain bread every day. Chicken was on his menu about five days a week. He drank orange juice, always freshly squeezed, daily. The only whole fruits he ate were apples and bananas, usually one of each a day. George had never really liked vegetables, but he did have two servings a day of broccoli, carrots, or cauliflower. Snacks, consumed every midday, were whole-grain crackers and cheddar cheese. His diet was supplemented with daily multivitamins and multiminerals.

As he responded to questions, it became obvious that George was probably suffering from food sensitivities. The principal reason for suspecting food sensitivities was the multiple symptoms he was experiencing involving his nervous system (depression), generalized unexplained aches and pains, fatigue, weight gain that did not respond to a low-calorie diet and exercise, his own and his family's history of allergies, his habits of limiting his diet to only a few foods that he ate over and over again, and the fact that his medical and laboratory examinations were always normal in spite of his complaints.

FOOD SENSITIVITIES DEFINED

Depending on which physician you talk to, you may come away with the idea that either there is no such thing as a food sensitivity or all human ills may be explained in terms of food sensitivities! Let's search for the truth between these two extremes.

The truth is many people, like George, have responded to regimens designed to treat food sensitivities. As in most areas of medicine there is no 100 percent cure rate, but the experience of thousands of patients is too great to ignore.

WHY DO FOOD SENSITIVITIES OCCUR?

No one really has the answer to that question, but there are a couple of interesting hypotheses. One suggestion is the digestive enzymes of the person with such sensitivities are not breaking down food properly. The consequence is that although foods are broken down into a size small enough to pass through the intestine into the blood, the particles are larger than the body expects. The immune system views the large particles as foreign objects and is triggered into action. The symptoms of a sensitivity reaction result from the body's attempts to attack those foreign substances.

Another hypothesis links the problem of larger particles with the physical condition of the intestines. If there are small injuries to the intestinal wall, possibly caused by yeast, the same scenario of large particles being absorbed and causing sensitivities could take place.

If food sensitivities are suspected, the detective work necessary for uncovering the offending foods doesn't have to be frustrating so long as it is approached logically, step-by-step. There are two ways to classify food sensitivities—they can be immediate or delayed. An immediate reaction may take place anywhere from several seconds to a few minutes after eating the offending food. It usually doesn't take many experiences to recognize the food causing the problem and take the appropriate therapeutic step: Avoid the food.

The second (and less easily diagnosable) type of reaction is a delayed reaction. The reaction might take place anywhere from a few hours to several hours after eating the food. Trying to identify the food is complicated by the time delay and by the fact that in delayed-reaction sensitivities several foods are usually involved.

The most important fact about delayed food sensitivities is that the trigger foods are usually eaten frequently, perhaps three or more times per week. They may in fact be some of your favorite foods. This immediately narrows down the foods to consider as possible offenders. In our society most people consume dairy products, grains (particularly wheat, rye, and rice), chicken, eggs, and beef several times a week. Most of the time it is not necessary to be concerned with rutabaga, turnips, or persimmons, for example, because these foods are not consumed frequently. If they were, however, then they, too, would become suspect.

UNCOVERING DELAYED FOOD SENSITIVITIES

There are many methods used to determine delayed food sensitivities. The two most common methods are food challenges and laboratory blood testing. Each method has advantages and disadvantages; no one method is universally accepted.

FOOD CHALLENGES

The idea behind food challenges is to see if the symptom in question can be brought on by eating a certain food. A warning is in order here. If the symptom is a serious one that may be dangerous, such as faintness, severe drop in blood pressure, or any loss of consciousness, the tests should be carried out by a qualified professional who is able to manage any possible emergency that may arise. Fortunately such symptoms are rare. Most symptoms fall into the classification of annoying and disturbing rather than life threatening.

A physician does the food testing in an office, most often by placing a few drops of varying dilutions of the food to be tested under the tongue and then observing the person for several minutes. The biggest disadvantages of this type of testing are that it is time-consuming and costly. Another problem is that the reaction to the food may not be the reaction being looked for. It may be subtle, such as a slight elevation in the pulse rate or slight changes in mood or behavior. The subtle changes may be significant, and for effective use of this method, the physician and his staff need to be experienced and to observe carefully.

Doing Food Challenges on Your Own

By following a few simple procedures, you can do food challenges by yourself and can gain much information. As mentioned earlier, a big part of the problem in identifying this type of food sensitivity is that the reaction is delayed. In food challenging, the first step is to convert the delayed reaction into an immediate reaction. This is done simply by staying away from that particular food for four days. The actual challenge is done by eating the food by itself according to the directions given below. With few exceptions, if there is a reaction to the food, it will take place within two hours. One exception is when testing dairy products and grains; if there is no reaction by the end of two hours, challenge again by eating the food being tested. If there is no reaction at the end of the second two-hour challenge, the food may be considered a nonreactor, or a nontrigger food.

CHALLENGING SINGLE FOODS

- Don't eat the suspected food for four days.
- If symptoms improve, eat the suspected food by itself on an empty stomach (at least two hours after previous meal).
- If there is a recurrence of symptoms, assume that you are sensitive to that food; it is a trigger food.
- Exception: When testing grain and dairy products, if there is no recurrence of symptoms, challenge with the same food again two hours later before assuming it is a nontrigger food.

Testing Multiple Foods with Challenging

The steps outlined above work well for testing one food at a time, but if multiple foods are suspected, there are some shortcuts you can take to avoid waiting four days between testing each food. Choose about three foods that you rarely eat, such as lamb, turnips, and papayas, and eat only those foods for four days. (Yes, this may sound "yucky" but it is better than fasting to cleanse your digestive tract.) Start the actual challenge on the fifth day, but only if there has been an improvement in your symptoms after manipulating your diet. If, for example, your main symptom has been headaches and after four days of limiting your diet to a few new foods the headaches have not improved, there is little sense in challenging foods, because the elimination of the foods did not result in an improvement. If, on the other hand, after eating the new (rarely chosen) foods for four days there has been a noticeable improvement, then your symptoms are probably food related and you can proceed with food challenging.

Challenge only one food at a time. If there has been no reaction at the end of the two hours (except for dairy products and grains as noted earlier), then the next food may be tested. If you have a reaction, then wait until all signs of this reaction have abated before you challenge the next food.

TESTING FOR MULTIPLE TRIGGER FOODS

- Choose three foods unusual to your diet.
- Eat only those three foods repeatedly for four days.
- If symptoms improve, proceed with food challenging.
- Make a list of foods that you eat regularly (three or more times a week); be especially suspicious of foods that you crave.
- Test by eating one different habitual food every two hours. If no reaction occurs, proceed to the next food challenge.
- If there is a reaction, be certain that all symptoms have cleared before going on to the next food.
- When testing a grain or dairy product, challenge again two hours later before considering it a nontrigger food.
- Keep a written diary of foods you have tested and your reactions to them to pinpoint trigger foods.

Here is an important hint. If a reaction occurs, it may last to a varying extent for four days. You can reduce a reaction to only a few hours if you ingest a combination of sodium bicarbonate and potassium bicarbonate at the first sign of the reaction. Don't try to mix the combination yourself; it has already been done for you. You'll find the combination in Alka-Seltzer in the gold foil, the brand labeled for use in relieving indigestion. Don't confuse this with the regular blue-foil Alka-Seltzer, which won't help reduce the food reactions at all. For those who prefer capsules, Klaire Laboratories (see appendix 1 for the address) distributes Bi-Carb Formula to health-food stores. Two Bi-Carb Formula capsules taken immediately after a reaction is noted will do the same as the two Alka-Seltzer gold-wrapped tablets.

LABORATORY TESTS FOR FOOD SENSITIVITIES

A special lab test screens the blood for evidence of an immune response to a particular food. The different immune complexes looked at are limited only by the amount of money available for testing. The tests involved are the immunoglobulin E (IgE) and immunoglobulin G (IgG).

The immediate food reactions are most often found in the IgE group, and the delayed food reactions are most often found in the IgG group. As mentioned previously, the immediate reactions carry very little mystery or difficulty in diagnosis. It is the delayed reactions that test the patience of the physician and client alike.

The IgG reactions comprise four subgroups, IgG1, IgG2, etc. Some laboratories suggest that the delayed reactions are found only in IgG4, others suggest that any of the four subgroups may be involved in delayed food reactions. Because there is a question about which subgroups are most significant, it is probably safest to test for as many of the subgroups as possible.

The number of foods that can be tested by looking at the IgG reactions is limitless. Usually it is best to test for all the foods you eat several times a week, any foods you feel you crave, plus several other foods not eaten as frequently. The idea is not only to identify the foods that are causing a reaction, but also to identify foods that are safest to eat while you withdraw from the problem foods.

The cytotoxic test, another blood test, also tests for sensitivity to an unlimited number of foods. The test is valid only if an experienced technician performs it, because scoring of the test results depends on the technician's ability to identify damaged white blood cells correctly after those cells have been mixed with the food substance being tested. Because the scoring is subjective, rather than objective machine scoring, the test is highly questionable in the minds of many who license its use. As a result, this test, which has proven very helpful when done by responsible technicians, is no longer generally available.

Another laboratory blood test is RAST (radioallergosorbent test). Its effectiveness is limited by the small variety of foods that can be tested by this method. Scratch tests, which involve placing extracts of food on the skin with a needle and looking for a reaction, are done frequently. Often, the results do not contribute much useful information, especially compared to some of the other less-intrusive tests. Another clinical test that is informative is the injection of varying doses of food extracts under the skin; the physician then looks for a swelling at the site of the injection. Although this method is useful in uncovering food sensitivities, its major drawbacks are the time and expense of doing the tests. Only a few of these tests can be done on the same day because it takes time for a "wheal" to form on the site, showing a definite reaction.

In summary, doing food challenges on your own may be a good option if you suspect only a few trigger foods, if there are constraints on the amount of money you can spend on testing, or if laboratory facilities are not available. (Some of the IgG testing may be done in laboratories not in your immediate community through the use of overnight express couriers.) Laboratory tests for IgG reactions are useful if multiple trigger foods are suspected, which are cumbersome to test by challenging.

TREATMENT OF FOOD SENSITIVITIES

Once you have identified your trigger foods, the best treatment involves simply eliminating those foods. Whenever possible, do not consume any food in your diet more than once in four days. By not repeating foods, you are doing some good preventive work—you won't develop a whole new set of trigger foods!

The Mood-Control Diet is an excellent program to follow. Don't repeat any food in a four-day cycle. After four months, about 95 percent of the foods that were your original trigger foods will no longer be reactive. They may be gradually reintroduced into your diet, but be careful not to repeat any food more than once every four days. The 4-day Rotation Plan that follows is an example of how you may pattern the Mood-Control Diet to avoid the repetition of any single food within a four-day period.

4-DAY FOOD-ROTATION PLAN

FIRST DAY

Breakfast

> Sliced orange or orange juice
> Rye flatbread (no wheat)
> Peanut butter

Lunch

> Filet of sole, flounder, or codfish
> Carrots
> Celery
> Sliced pineapple

Dinner

> Cooked artichoke or canned artichoke hearts
> Broiled lamb chop or sliced lamb roast
> Acorn squash, hubbard squash, mashed cooked pumpkin, or
>   melon
> Spinach
> Apricots

SECOND DAY

Breakfast

Blueberries
2 eggs, boiled, poached, or scrambled in safflower oil

Lunch

Canned salmon, fresh salmon, or tuna packed in water
Lettuce
Broiled or sliced tomato
Banana

Dinner

Broiled chicken or roast duck
Baked potato
Broccoli, Brussels sprouts, or cauliflower
Pear halves

THIRD DAY

Breakfast

½ grapefruit
Cottage cheese, yogurt, or other cheese or milk product

Lunch

Shrimp, clams, lobster, mussels, scallops, or haddock
Rice
Peas, green beans, lima beans, or chick-peas
Sliced peaches, plums, or nectarines

Dinner

Beef or veal patties, or cooked plain sliced beef or veal
Onions and mushrooms sautéed in corn oil
Corn
Zucchini or crookneck yellow squash
Strawberries

FOURTH DAY

Breakfast

> Cranberry juice
> Oatmeal cereal (no milk), pure wheat cereal (no milk), or wheat
>   toast with raspberry jam

Lunch

> Sliced turkey with natural gravy
> Asparagus
> Beets
> Figs

Dinner

> Pork chops, pork roast, baked bass or red snapper
> Baked sweet potato
> Cabbage, green or red
> Baked apple or applesauce

BEWARE OF FOOD FAMILY MEMBERS

Sometimes foods in the same family are so similar—like identical twins—
that if one of the foods is a trigger food, the others in the family should be
placed high on your list of suspected trigger foods as well. At other times,
however, even foods in the same family are so divergent that it is not
necessary to eliminate all of them just because one of them triggers a
reaction.

The food family members so closely related that they may be considered identical twins are

- Beef, veal, and dairy products from cow's milk
- Chicken eggs and chicken
- Wheat and rye

When confronted with an identical twin sensitivity situation, it is
advisable to do a food challenge within that food family to determine
which members may cause a reaction (see appendix 2).

Trigger foods should be eliminated for a minimum period of four months. At the end of that time, if there has been symptomatic improvement, the foods may be reintroduced into the diet and eaten no more than once in every four days. Generally, about 95 percent of the foods that were reactive will no longer be so and will stay unreactive as long as they are not eaten more frequently than once in every four days. Reintroduce each trigger food at least one week apart.

SUGGESTED SUPPLEMENT PROGRAM

People with multiple food sensitivities may be deprived of important nutrients. Some supplementation can provide insurance of optimal health despite a limited variety of foods. Be sure to discuss this with your physician.
- *Basic.* Nonallergenic (read the label) multivitamin and mineral. Follow the recommended dosage on the product you select.
- *Specific.* A mixed digestive enzyme including hydrochloric acid and pancreatic enzymes (available in health-food stores) is sometimes helpful. The hydrochloric acid supplement should not be taken by anyone who produces excessive acid or who has any history of ulceration occurring in the upper gastrointestinal tract, the esophagus, stomach, or duodenum (the small intestine leading from the stomach). Belching or flatulence may be signals of such excessive acid.

As mentioned earlier, a mixture of sodium bicarbonate and potassium bicarbonate, as found in Alka-Seltzer in the gold foil or Bi-Carb Formula, taken immediately after recognizing a food reaction will limit the symptoms to a few hours.

Sometimes a combination of quercetin, part of the vitamin C complex, and bromelain, a digestive enzyme derived from pineapple (available from Optimum Health Labs, see appendix 1 for their address), taken about thirty minutes before meals can help modify any sensitivity reaction. Again, follow the dosage directions on the labels of the products. This preparation is particularly helpful if you have so many sensitivities that you cannot eliminate or rotate all the foods; it is also helpful if it is not possible to identify all the foods that trigger your reactions.

TO OVERCOME FOOD SENSITIVITIES

- Find your trigger food(s) by
  - Physician's testing/lab testing.

– Personal food challenging.
* When you have found your trigger food(s)
  –Carefully eliminate them from your diet.
  –Study the 4-Day Food-Rotation Plan to learn how to rotate food choices.
  –Follow the Mood-Control Diet, always rotating choices of foods. Make your own modifications to eliminate your trigger food(s), or if tolerable, rotate such food every four days.
  –Use the recipes in part II, noting which ones are free of your trigger food(s)—all the recipes are marked (dairy-free, egg-free, gluten-free, sugar-free, or yeast-free) and if substitutions can be made, that notation accompanies each recipe as well.
* Refer to appendix 2 to determine the biological relationships of your trigger food(s); avoid related foods that could cause problems.

5

YEAST: WHEN FRIEND BECOMES FOE

Yeast organisms and the related molds and fungi are found throughout nature. Most of the time these organisms are helpful and they enrich many diets. Bread without yeast is a hard cracker. But when the yeast gets where it doesn't belong, the host of this otherwise helpful organism could be in for trouble.

In the 1970s, C. Orian Truss, M.D., a practicing physician in Birmingham, Alabama, gave one of his female patients a dose of an antiyeast medication to combat a vaginal yeast infection, which occurred during the course of treatment for another condition. After a short time, the patient reported something startling: Her long-standing conditions of depression and mental confusion started to clear up after taking the antiyeast medication. Over the next several months, Dr. Truss continued to note a connection between yeast infections and healthy brain function as manifested by mood, mental acuity, memory, and clarity of thought.

Dr. Truss's studies spanned several more years of clinical observations and were reported at medical meetings, in medical journals, and, finally, in his book *The Missing Diagnosis*.

Candidiasis, as the condition is named, is a sensitivity to *Candida albicans*, a yeast organism that frequently infects a human host. It is important to emphasize that this condition is not a generalized yeast infection. A generalized yeast infection occurs only in those people who have a severely compromised immune system, either through a long-standing debilitating illness or through the use of medications that are intended to neutralize the immune system. A generalized yeast infection is life threatening and is *not* what we are talking about here. The condition we are discussing is a common, but often unrecognized, condition. It is not life threatening and does not become life threatening, although it does compromise the quality of life to a significant degree when it is present and undiagnosed.

Candida grows easily, and once it is present it is difficult to eliminate. Moist surfaces are preferred, so it grows well in the vagina, the gastrointestinal tract, and the respiratory system. The yeast grows on the surface of the tissue, and that is where part of the problem starts. By establishing

33

itself on the surface of the tissue, it has also established itself in an area virtually unreached by the immune system. Until the yeast actually invades the superficial tissue, where it can be dealt with by the immune system, it is free to multiply and it does. After yeast proliferates, the host has a hard time ridding itself of the fungus. Recurrent infections quickly become the rule rather than the exception.

The long-standing problem with *Candida* occurs because during the life cycle of *Candida* there is a time when products from the yeast are excreted into the superficial tissue of the host. A host with an intact immune system starts to fight off those products, which are foreign to it. After repeated attacks, however, a sensitivity to those yeast products can develop.

THE THREE-LEVEL SYMPTOMS PATTERN OF YEAST

Yeast sensitivity reveals itself in three levels of symptoms. The first level is the target organ's response. The target organs are usually the nervous system, resulting in a dysfunction manifested by thinking difficulty and mood changes, and in women, the endocrine system, resulting in irregular menses and/or changes of flow. The second level is a localized group of symptoms which vary depending on where the yeast is proliferating: the gastrointestinal tract, the vagina, or pulmonary system. The third level of problems is caused because the yeast sensitivity sets the stage for increased food and inhalant sensitivities which may result in a variety of symptoms.

Target organs are those organs affected by a sensitivity. For example, if you developed a skin rash after eating strawberries, the target organ would be the skin. The organ system that seems most often vulnerable to sensitivities is the nervous system, particularly the brain. When this occurs, the function of the brain, including thinking and mood, becomes disordered. Patients complain of depression for which they cannot find an adequate psychological explanation. Thinking is muddled, concentration and memory are poor, and the logical progression of thoughts is disturbed; people report feeling unable to make decisions. Needless to say this can wreak havoc with career and relationships.

In women, the endocrine system is often a target organ. Menstruation may become irregular and flow may be abnormally heavy or light.

The second level of symptoms relates to the location of the *Candida* growth. An overgrowth of yeast in the vagina is easily recognized as a white "cottage cheese" discharge. Gastrointestinal symptoms may extend from the mouth and throat, which will exhibit white patches on the mucous membrane, to bloating after eating, alternating diarrhea and constipation, and itching around the anus. Respiratory problems may include hoarseness, shortness of breath, chronic cough, and asthma.

The third level of symptoms results from yeast sensitivity, promoting the development of food and inhalant sensitivities. These sensitivities may be responsible for many other symptoms. Any food sensitivity may affect any organ in the system as a target organ. Inhalants may also be a problem. For some reason, those with Candidiasis are often particularly sensitive to perfumes and to smog.

CANDIDA INFECTIONS

Although vaginal yeast sometimes begins to grow after intercourse, the yeast problem is not solely caused by sexual intercourse. The principal conditions that favor yeast growth are a high-carbohydrate diet, particularly those diets high in refined carbohydrates (yeast thrives on sugars and starches); the use of antibiotics (they knock out the good bacteria in the intestines), especially the broad spectrum antibiotics such as the tetracycline family; and high progesterone blood levels that occur during pregnancy, during the premenstrual stage, and when taking birth control pills. It is easy to see how the medical profession has been an unknowing accomplice in allowing the spread of this damaging yeast disorder. Birth control pills and antibiotics are freely prescribed; sometimes they are necessary, but sometimes they are not.

Ruth's case is a good example of how problems can be perpetuated and complicated when the diagnosis of candidiasis is overlooked. When she first met Dr. Ross, Ruth was a thirty-seven-year-old, single woman who was holding an executive position in one of the major movie studios. Her on-again, off-again relationship with her live-in boyfriend, Leo, was off-again when she first consulted Dr. Ross. In evaluating her depression—the principal reason for her consultation—it was quickly apparent that her depression had been long-standing, at various degrees of intensity, and that her breakup with Leo, which followed a fairly regular pattern of about twice a year, may have been responsible for the recent increase in her symptoms, but it could not have been responsible for similar symptoms that had been present for many years. It seemed there was more to her depression than her unsatisfying relationship.

Ruth's other long-standing symptoms included fatigue and general lack of well-being, bloating after eating, some diarrhea as well as constipation, and an embarrassing anal itch. She began to experience some joint pains, mostly in the joints of her right hand, but there were also hip and back pains. The symptoms seemed to be with her at all times, but not to the same degree. For example, during her premenstrual phase she always experienced worse symptoms. Ruth was almost philosophical about adding premenstrual syndrome (PMS) to her already extensive list of complaints. Another problem didn't surprise her.

Ruth suspected that all the discord she had been having with Leo was not only due to his problems, which she chronicled to him in great detail when they argued. Her lack of sexual drive over the past few years had added another source of tension to their relationship. She realized that they hadn't had an evening away from the apartment in about three months because she always felt so exhausted after work that she wanted to rest in bed. They hadn't been away for a long camping weekend, an activity they both had enjoyed, for over a year. Ruth's guilt, once she was aware that her problems were contributing to the troubled relationship, was difficult for her to handle, but it also was one of the underlying strong motivations for her agreeing to seek further help when her family doctor suggested it.

When Dr. Ross questioned her closely about the onset of her problems, Ruth recalled with some surprise that the last time in her life when she had really felt well was about the age of twenty. At that time she had had a serious bout of appendicitis, requiring an operation and a long course of antibiotics. She also remembered, when questioned, that she began to develop vaginal yeast infections around that time and that the first one occurred in the hospital. The infections cleared promptly with treatment, but they also recurred frequently over the next four to five years. She then went through a time when she had yeast infections no more than twice a year, but she was concerned about her irregular menstrual periods. Her physician put her on birth control pills; however, as Ruth's periods became more regular, she began to experience more yeast infections. Even though she was taken off the birth control pills (after developing a severe skin eruption, which was treated with antibiotics), she noticed an increase of symptoms over the next several years, from about the time she was thirty-one. By the time she arrived in Dr. Ross's office, she stated that although she was thirty-seven, she felt seventy-seven.

After obtaining the history of her illness, Dr. Ross ordered a blood test to check Ruth's immunological response to *Candida*. The test confirmed the suspected diagnosis and treatment for *Candida* infection was started. After about one week she thought she felt better, but her observations were vague. After about eight weeks, she reported Leo had moved back in and they were enjoying themselves as they had when they first met. They were going out a few nights a week and had gone away on a long weekend, which they both enjoyed.

As she improved over the next several months, Ruth noticed that she experienced some irritability and mild abdominal complaints whenever she ate wheat. She stopped wheat entirely and noticed further improvement. After about one year, she forgot to take her medication on a business trip and within one week began to experience some of her old physical and mental symptoms again. Resuming her medication quickly eliminated the symptoms.

Everything has worked out well for Ruth and continues to do so as long as she follows her treatment program. At first she found the treatment program cumbersome and resented the time and attention it took. After a few months, however, she became an enthusiastic participant, because, as she told Dr. Ross, she was seeing something good and she was feeling good too—better than she had in years. She is looking forward to the time when she can be a little less vigilant about her diet and medication, but she willingly follows her special program because she knows that her best chances of staying well come with a continued program for two or three years.

A TWO-PRONGED ATTACK ON YEAST

There are two main lines of treatment for candidiasis. The first is through the use of medication, some ancillary nutritional products, and yeast-free vitamins and minerals. Nystatin has been used for many years and is one of the few prescription medications that is not accompanied by a long list of frightening side effects. The only side effect noted by the manufacturer is possible gastrointestinal upsets with large doses. This side effect can sometimes be avoided if the outer covering of the generic nystatin is soaked in water for twenty minutes and the coating scraped off. The reaction seems to be from a sensitivity to the color and coating of the tablet rather than to the nystatin itself. This reaction may also be avoided by using pure nystatin powder, available in some pharmacies in bulk form or in gelatin capsules. The other side effect experienced with nystatin occurs because the drug kills the *Candida* organisms. The kill off of the yeast releases into the body the same material that the system is allergic to. This causes a temporary increase in symptoms. Because of this kill-off effect, nystatin is usually started at a low dosage, which is increased after four days. In about 10 to 15 percent of cases there is no kill off at the low dosage, but the kill off occurs at the higher dosage. When this happens, the higher dosage can be initially reduced and then increased gradually to its highest level.

Another useful nutritional product is acidophilus. These good bacteria reside in the gastrointestinal tract, where they do many helpful things, one of which is to fight *Candida*. Antibiotics that are prescribed to fight infections (such as the recurrent yeast infections that Ruth had) and perhaps even trace amounts of antibiotics in our food supply (added to animal and poultry feed) quickly kill off these helpful organisms, so it is advisable to resupply them with supplementation, especially if you have been taking antibiotics or birth control pills. The pill increases progesterone levels, which provides a good environment for yeast growth. Acidophilus is available in health-food stores and should be kept in the refrigerator.

Garlic is also reputed to have antiyeast properties. To avoid the socially unacceptable odor of fresh garlic and pills, an odorless garlic capsule is the supplement of choice. This is available in health-food stores. The usual dosage for garlic capsules is two capsules, two or three times a day.

There are other nonprescription products marketed as yeast fighters, some of which are effective in certain cases. The most effective treatment, however, is the old standby, nystatin. More powerful antiyeast medications are available, but they are not satisfactory for candidiasis because of the increased possibility of serious side effects (such as liver damage) when using them over a prolonged period of time.

General nutritional supplements, such as multivitamin and mineral complexes, ensure that you receive needed nutrients. Nothing works right if the necessary nutrients are not present in the proper amounts. Any supplements taken by candidiasis sufferers should be yeast-free—read the labels!

The second line of treatment is dietary. The Mood-Control Diet, with special modifications for yeast dieters, is well balanced and will help you maintain optimal health while coping with ridding your body of yeast problems. Each week of menu plans has guidelines for this specific problem to make it easier for you to dine at home or in restaurants. In addition, the recipes in part II marked both sugar-free and yeast-free offer plenty of delicious choices. A dietary program is necessary for two reasons. First, all foods on which yeast feeds and proliferates must be removed from the diet. These include all sugars (including honey), enriched refined white flour, and quick-cooking refined white rice. The use of artificial sweeteners is discouraged, even though yeast does not feed on them. It is preferable to retrain your taste buds to avoid sweet-tasting food. After six weeks, if you are not under increased stress, which may cause a sugar craving, sugar will prove to be too sweet and therefore will be easy to avoid.

Fruits should be restricted to two servings a day (see chapter 10) because of the fructose (simple sugar) content of fruit.

The second reason for restricting your diet is to avoid all foods that you suspect you are sensitive to. If you have candidiasis, it is assumed, based on experience, that you are sensitive to all yeast and yeast-related products, molds, and fungi. Some clinicians will restrict all foods that may contain a mold or fungus. The list of forbidden foods then becomes large, and the more restrictive the diet, the more difficult it is to follow. Dr. Ross advises his patients to avoid only the most common foods abundant in yeast, mold, and fungus:

> Yeast (in baked goods such as bread, pastries, and cakes)
> Alcohol
> Vinegar
> Soy sauce (including tamari and teriyaki sauce)
> Moldy cheese (such as Roquefort, blue, and Limburger)
> Mushrooms

The most effective treatment of yeast sensitivity fights the yeast colonies on the two levels of medication and dietary manipulation. The use of nystatin, acidophilus, and yeast-free vitamins and minerals as well as a diet that avoids refined carbohydrates, limits fruits to two servings daily, and eliminates the yeast-containing foods noted above usually results in some positive effects within eight days of beginning the program (after the kill-off period when symptoms temporarily worsen). If some positive changes do not take place within the first twenty-one days and you have followed the program correctly, it would be wise to question the diagnosis.

MAKE A COMMITMENT TO STAYING WELL

The problem encountered most frequently in the management of this condition is that it is tempting to stop following the treatment plan once you begin to feel better. When the treatment becomes irregular, however, symptoms will return within about a week's time.

To beat *Candida* at its own game, certain parts of your treatment plan must be continued for two to three years. The important features of ongoing treatment are the continued use of the nystatin and the continued avoidance of refined carbohydrates (sugar, honey, syrups, and refined white flour). The yeast, mold, and fungus foods, which are initially restricted, may be reintroduced into your diet after four months' abstinence, but they should be tried only once you feel well and then consumed only once every four days maximum.

As time goes on, you will come to recognize a few important foods to which you are particularly sensitive. These foods should be eliminated for at least four months before gradual reintroduction into your diet. Follow the steps for detection and handling of food sensitivities in the previous chapter. As the fuel for your yeast sensitivity is removed, many of your previously unrecognized food sensitivities may also be diminished. Sometimes, however, certain food sensitivities seem to continue, especially if they have been well established over several years. In those instances, a direct investigation uncovering those sensitivities must be done. Undetected food sensitivities account for many of the treatment failures in candidiasis.

The good news is yeast sensitivity, for the most part, is treatable and the results can be excellent, restoring a good quality of life after delivering a knockout blow to the invaders.

6

HOW FOOD JUNKIES PAY THE PIPER

D R. ROSS SEES A SURPRISING NUMBER OF people who suffer from chronic depression and fatigue, who are simply suffering from the effects of poor food choices and poor eating habits. Their dogs and cats may eat impressively labeled, nutrition-packed, canned and dried food developed by Ph.D.'s in animal science. Such nourishment assures the owner that the animal will have good muscle tone, lustrous fur, the energy to get through the day with reasonable fitness, and the ability to live as long as possible. The human animal needs equal care!

If quality nourishment is missing from your diet there are telltale signs. Lack of energy, poor concentration and thinking, pessimistic attitudes, droopy hair, breaking nails, and unexplained skin problems are tip-offs to an imbalance of nutrients and/or poor absorption of vitamins and minerals essential to your looking good and feeling great.

If your problem is not caused by hypoglycemia, food sensitivities, or yeast infections, it may be attributed to how, when, and where you eat.

NUTRITION STRAIGHT TALK

Busy people—young, old, or in-between—often sacrifice proper meals for a variety of reasons, ranging from not being certain of the right foods to eat to being too busy to prepare a "square" meal. We hope that by the time you finish this book, you will know how important—and how easy—it is to eat right and feel right.

Busy people in the fast lane often satisfy hunger by snacking through-out the day, hitting a fast-food restaurant, or preparing meals from additive-loaded convenience foods. This results in a diet high in fats, hidden salt, and sugar and low in fresh fruits and vegetables. Long-term subnutrition robs the body of vital nutrients and results in a general sense of emotional and physical malaise.

On one level our bodies are magnificent factories, using raw material to build the chemicals needed to support the numerous functions that keep us going. Our bodies are constantly growing and repairing. To fulfill these functions, waste materials have to be efficiently removed, cells rapidly repaired, and foods have to be broken down to the basic chemical components that keep the body working well. A healthy body controls these functions to prevent overactivity or underactivity of any particular chemical reaction that, if allowed to occur, would result in disease.

Our blood carries a variety of hormones that control the occurrence and rate of all of these reactions. All the nutrients that the body uses are found in the bloodstream. If there is an overabundance or scarcity of these necessary nutrients, illness is the end result. The illness may be severe, but it often happens subtly: You may feel a general lack of well-being, have a depressed outlook, and have poor energy—all of which combine to prevent you from joining in and being part of the mainstream of life. When you don't feel well, life may not end, but it has a tendency to pass you by. Sometimes illness cannot be avoided, but more often it can. Avoiding illness and reaching for optimum health starts with supplying the basic materials the body needs, and that is within the reach of each of us when we sit down at every meal.

To be in charge of your daily diet, it's important to understand why a wide variety of foods is necessary in a well-balanced diet. There are several classes of nutrients: some are food types, others are vitamins and minerals. The basic food types are fats, proteins, and carbohydrates.

Fats include butter, margarine, oils, mayonnaise, lard, and meat fat. Fats provide a reserve of energy for the body.

Protein is found mainly in meat, poultry, eggs, fish, cheese, and other dairy products. Good-quality protein may also be obtained by combining a grain (rice, corn, pasta, or bread) with a legume (beans, peas, or nuts) at the same meal. Protein provides the building blocks of the body.

Carbohydrates are the sugars and starches. Simple carbohydrates, such as sugar, syrup, and honey are quickly converted to energy by the body. Complex carbohydrates, such as fruits, vegetables, and grains, are metabolized into energy more slowly and evenly and are a more desirable form of carbohydrate for that reason. Fiber found in some vegetables, fruits, and grains may be classed as a basic food type, although fiber provides bulk rather than nutrients.

These food types allow the body to renew energy and repair itself; vitamins and minerals are also necessary parts of the enzymatic reactions of building and repairing. Without the proper amounts of all of these nutrients, the work of keeping the body in a healthy state is impaired.

For the most part, the body is very forgiving. Although the nutrients outlined above are needed for proper functioning, it is unnecessary to have every nutrient at every meal. The body hoards nutrients for its own rainy days. Some nutrients are more easily stored than others. For example, vitamins A, D, E, and K are stored in the fat of the body, and vitamins B and C are water soluble and are not stored as easily because the body eliminates them via urine. Even so, people have survived fasts of more than sixty days without food before the body ran out of nutrients to sustain life. No one need be unusually concerned if an occasional day is a nutritional "wasteland." Problems begin to develop, however, when there is a long-standing lack of adequate nutrients being supplied to the body.

For many busy people, a typical day's diet may consist of grabbing some orange juice, coffee, and roll for breakfast; a quick club sandwich and coffee for lunch; a candy bar to revive failing energy in midafternoon; and a drink or two after work followed by a frozen dinner or a fast-food hamburger. A repetitious diet leads to deficiencies of vitamins or minerals or an imbalance of food types—usually too much fat, too much protein, too much simple carbohydrates from junk food, and too few of the complex carbohydrates that provide sustained energy as well as a wide variety of vitamins and minerals for the body's well-being.

A poor diet may also result in excess weight. The body has a tendency to store and hoard what it gets when it recognizes that it is not getting all that it needs. The net result is an overweight, but undernourished, person. The overweight person may further encourage the hoarding habit of the body by restricting calories and nutrients in an effort to lose weight. In the overall scheme of things, there are good and bad ways of accomplishing goals, and so it goes with weight loss. Fast weight loss is terrific if you need to lose five to ten pounds in a week to finish shooting a movie, have photographs taken for your modeling portfolio, or get into a suit or dress for the super social event of the season, but it's important to remember that weight lost in this way doesn't stay off.

It is difficult to scan the bestseller book lists without finding a weight-loss book hovering right up there near the top. These books sell well because so many people eat poorly, become overweight, and don't like it. These diet books fail their readers because most are focused on weight loss, rather than on attaining and maintaining proper weight and nutrient balance. The diet plans in most of these books could not be maintained indefinitely, because they do not provide proper nutrition.

The body is forgiving for a while, but not forever. When you attain your desired weight and then return to a "maintenance" diet—usually the way you were eating before you started the weight loss diet—most of the weight returns, sometimes with an unwanted bonus. The best way to lose weight permanently and safely is to eat a diet that is nutritious and correct for your body's metabolism. Everyone has individual nutritional needs, but an overconsumption of fats and sugar-laden foods is bound to end up as fat on your body. The best way to lose weight is to eat the right foods and be patient. Excess poundage is rarely accumulated over a short period of time and it won't come off and stay off if you try the latest fad diet. Slow and steady is the way to go. A successful weight loss may amount to as much as three pounds a week for the first two weeks. After that, be happy with a loss of a pound a week. Rapid weight loss is rarely permanent weight loss and can be a shock to the body.

This is why the problem of weight loss extends beyond the simple formula of the difference between calories in and calories out. There are some people who have perfectly working hormonal systems who will diet and still not be able to lose as much weight as they should. They may, in fact, not be able to lose any weight at all. Others have the experience of losing very little on a very strict diet and are upset and mystified when they put on several pounds overnight after they eat a little extra something such as a piece of bread or cake (they are allergic to wheat and don't know it). Research has shown that people with this kind of weight problem experience fluid retention from eating foods to which their bodies are sensitive. When these people discover the hidden allergies and follow a rotary diet such as the one outlined in chapter 4, they often find that weight loss becomes a much simpler matter than they have ever experienced.

A special problem that has received attention in the last few years is an eating disorder known as bulimia. Bulimia is uncontrollable eating, usually gorging of unbelievable proportions. In one sitting, a person suffering with this malady could easily consume a whole cake, a loaf of bread, several candy bars, a few quarts of milk topped off with two quarts of ice cream. This illness occurs most often in young women, who hide the malady. They don't usually gain weight because they take laxatives and/or induce vomiting after they've eaten, so the food doesn't have time to be absorbed.

The other part of this syndrome is known as anorexia nervosa. An anorexic person may go for weeks or months with minimal food intake. This phenomenon is usually suffered by young women who are dissatisfied with their body images. Even when they are skin and bones, they still perceive themselves to be overweight. Teenagers may suffer from anorexia because of a fear of growing up and having to cope with sexuality, which is manifested in their developing bodies. A young anorexic woman becomes psychologically fixated on achieving a skinny preadolescent figure. Often this results in loss of menstrual periods and body weights that reach lows of eighty to ninety pounds. Eventually a medical emergency arises because the lack of nutrients becomes life threatening. Bulimia and anorexia are complicated problems involving both physical and psychological elements. Whatever the cause, the effect is devastating to proper body and mental functioning, and it can take years to overcome the damage of these syndromes.

Underweight is a major cause of death around the world, and should be regarded as a dangerous practice if the diet is so limited in nutrient intake that the body's functions are diminished or impaired. Lean optimum weight is a desirable goal, but it should never be reached by malnutrition and it should always be in line with reasonable expectations for your age, sex, and body type, which your doctor can easily clarify. It is important to have realistic perceptions of your body image and to understand the role that a wide variety of nutrients plays in preserving your health.

NUTRITION "GOOD GUYS" AT A GLANCE

It is simple to define good nutrition as a dietary intake that supplies all of the essential nutrients in quantities necessary for optimum function. But what does that mean for the individual? No one except yourself is going to be able to tell you what is the best diet for you (unless you are ill in which case you and your doctor agree on a proper dietary regimen). Different people's biochemistries are as different as their facial features. No nutritional guru or wise university professor can devise a diet that is perfect for everyone. Each individual must discover his or her own formula for dietary success.

To do this, you need specific information. In gathering this information, be critical. There is much disagreement about proper nutrition because all the facts aren't yet known. Basically, however, there are two general schools of thought to be aware of.

University nutrition departments tend to find no fault with what might be called the average American diet comprising many foods developed in food-processing plants and served in fast-food restaurants. They generally hold that the average American diet provides sufficient nutrients to maintain normal health and that no vitamin or mineral supplements are necessary.

Opposed to this group are a large number of physicians and nutritionists who use nutrition as a primary tool to deal with health and disease. This group of healers and a significant portion of the general population believe the average American diet has been robbed of its vitality by processing and, because of the poor food choices people have been led to make, it has become dangerous to health. They advocate a return to unprocessed food wherever possible and usually endorse the generous use of supplements. As with most things, the truth probably lies somewhere between the extremes.

In defense of some food processing, it should be obvious that we could live without processing only in a strictly agricultural community. Our society, with its large cities, which are sometimes very distant from agricultural centers, requires that some foods be frozen or canned to reach all areas of the population. Without processing, populations might suffer from malnutrition to a more marked degree than with processing.

The argument against some kinds of processing is directed toward the large numbers of chemicals added to foods. Some of these additives, which are numbered in the thousands, have had to undergo strict tests for safety. However, there are hundreds of chemicals added to foods that have not been tested but are allowed and categorized as GRAS (generally regarded as safe), because they have been used for such a long time. There is a question of the true safety of the large group of GRAS additives.

Another criticism of processed foods is the use of artificial foods, those that have been entirely manufactured to look like and taste like the real thing. It has become possible through modern technology to sit down to a meal that is entirely man-made. Concern has been expressed about the long-term effects of consuming large amounts of these foods on a regular basis.

The problem of processing is not whether or not it should exist. It does and it will, because it is necessary. The problem is our lack of understanding about how processing may be undermining our health and how to compensate for it by using fresh foods and nutritional supplements.

The first step in making food choices is to be aware that each of the food types—protein, fats, and carbohydrates—is necessary in proper balance and quantity. Each type has its good guys and bad guys. Let's review them.

PROTEIN

Protein is needed to build and repair the body. It may be obtained from animal and nonanimal sources. Proteins are made up of building blocks called amino acids. There are hundreds of amino acids, most of which can be synthesized in the body from even smaller chemical groups. However, there are a few essential amino acids that can be obtained only from eating protein, because the human body cannot manufacture them. Not only must those essential amino acids be supplied from outside the body, they must be eaten in the proper proportions to be efficiently used. In nature, the only source of these essential amino acids in the proper proportion is found in meat (this includes fish and poultry). If you do not eat meat, these essential amino acids may still be found in foods such as legumes and grains, but these foods must be combined in specific ways to deliver all of the amino acids at the same time for the body's use. Natives of many cultures combine beans and corn or beans and rice in the same dish to provide high-quality protein that includes the essential amino acids. Eating these foods at separate meals does not provide the same effect.

Eggs and dairy products deliver all essential amino acids on their own, but we do not usually consume these in sufficient quantities to fill our protein needs. Combining them with legumes and grains provides additional protein. This can often produce a nutritious protein that is less expensive than meat, fish, or poultry. Protein should comprise about 12 percent of the total calories of your daily menu to provide the essential amino acids needed for building and repairing your body.

FATS

Basically, fats fall into the hard or solid fats, called "saturated" (animal-source fats) and the liquid fats, "unsaturated" (vegetable-source fats). Fats are essential for proper functioning and are the basic molecules of many hormones that regulate the occurrence and tempo of the body's processes.

There is current agreement within the medical profession and among nutritionists concerning the role that fat plays in illness, especially in the development of fat plaques inside the arteries, which interfere with blood flow and put people at risk for heart attacks and strokes. Nutritional surveys of the American diet reveal a high proportion of calories derived from saturated fat and a lower proportion from unsaturated fats. The unsaturated fats or oils prepared by a process known as "cold pressing" retain the nutrient value of the oil. Liquid oils processed by other means subject the nuts or seeds to high temperatures, resulting in the destruction of many of the nutrients found in the oils in the natural state.

Polyunsaturated oils tend to lower the amount of low density lipoprotein (LDL), a blood component that produces fat deposits in the arteries, but they also lower high density lipoprotein (HDL), a beneficial component that aids in eliminating cholesterol from the blood.

Lately, nutritionists are paying more attention to monounsaturated fats found in such fish as salmon, tuna, and mackerel. These contain omega-3 fatty acids, which have been found to lower LDL while maintaining a higher HDL. Olive oil and canola oil, high in monounsaturated fat, are also good sources of omega-6 fatty acids. Recent studies indicate that monounsaturated oils play a greater role than polyunsaturated oil in regulating blood cholesterol levels. This is why eating monounsaturated oils is preferable to consuming the polyunsaturated oils.

Understand that some fat in the diet is essential. Generally, it is wise to divide your intake of fat into thirds, with one-third coming from animal fat (fat grained in well-trimmed meat, egg yolks, butter, cheese, and whole milk), one-third coming from polyunsaturated fat (vegetable oils such as corn oil, safflower oil, and sunflower oil) and the final one-third from monounsaturated fat (fish oil, olive oil, and canola oil). It is wise to limit your total fat intake to 20 to 30 percent of your total calories of each day.

For a better understanding of the categories of fat sources, here is a quick guide to those most often used. Note that cholesterol is found only in the animal-source fats, but that coconut oil and palm oil, although from vegetable sources, are exceptionally high in saturated fat. These are the oils most often used in cookies, candy, and other sweet treats. Watch for them in ingredient listings and steer clear of them whenever you can.

QUICK GUIDE TO DIETARY FATS

Fat	Cholesterol mg/tbsp	Saturated Fat (%)	Polyunsaturated Fat (%)	Monounsaturated Fat (%)
Canola Oil	0	6	36	58
Safflower Oil	0	9	78	13
Sunflower Oil	0	11	69	20
Corn Oil	0	13	62	25
Olive Oil	0	14	9	77
Soybean Oil	0	15	61	24
Peanut Oil	0	18	34	48
Cottonseed Oil	0	27	54	19
Lard	12	41	12	47
Palm Oil	0	51	10	39
Beef Fat	14	52	4	44
Butterfat	33	66	4	30
Coconut Oil	0	92	2	6

Source: USDA Human Nutrition Service

CARBOHYDRATES

There are definitely good guys and bad guys among foods that supply carbohydrates. Carbohydrates include vegetables, fruits, grains, and sugar. The good guys are the complex carbohydrates, such as fruits, whole grains, and vegetables. The bad guys are the simple sugars and refined grains.

In our diets, simple carbohydrates are usually overconsumed in the form of sugar, white flour, and white rice. These processed carbohydrates provide only the carbohydrate molecule, but carry no vitamins or minerals with them. In order for the body to utilize the carbohydrate, the vitamins and minerals must be supplied from another source. The problem is that carbohydrates reduce your appetite for other foods, which results in relative vitamin and mineral deficiencies when large amounts of these processed foods are eaten. Processed carbohydrates are also low in fiber, which is important for proper digestive mechanisms and better colon functioning.

A whole grain, in contrast, supplies not only carbohydrates but also protein, vitamins, minerals, and fiber. The main value of processing (removing the outer layers of grains) is that the processed grain may be stored without rotting and with limited danger of insect infestation. Insects do not seem to find the processed, devitalized grain very appealing. If the processed white flour doesn't appeal to the self-preserving instincts of insects, what value do you suppose it has for you?

There is an art to selecting foods that will enhance your energy, mood, and well-being. Processed foods and many fast foods just don't deliver what your body needs. As nutrients are digested and absorbed, they are converted by biochemical action into usable energy, into storage depots as triglycerides, or into amino acid building blocks.

Everything you eat goes to work, to storage for future reconversion to energy, or to waste. If you select a wide variety of foods, you give your body the abundance of vitamins and minerals needed for every step of its actions and reactions. If the food you select is stripped of nutrients or if you eat a lot of the same foods, you may consume a lot of calories and yet be malnourished.

If you take in extra carbohydrates, some of what isn't used for glucose is stored in muscle tissue as glycogen. The rest is stored as triglycerides in the fatty warehouses of your body—on your hips, waist, stomach, and thighs. There it is joined by the overflow of your protein and fat intake. Your body seems to be designed to save calories for a rainy day, week, or month. The trouble is, in this land of plenty, extra triglycerides are banked daily, yet there is often no need to draw on this energy account. Biochemically, once food is stored as triglycerides, it can only be converted back into glucose. A new supply of protein must be eaten every day to keep the body in good repair.

The object of the nutrition game is to eat smart, take in a generous supply of nutrients and calories for your biochemical needs, store just enough so that you never run out of energy, but not so much that you become a walking warehouse of triglycerides. There is no sense in adding to your fat collection if you already have enough! Below is a guide to help you make wise food selections.

QUICK GUIDE TO HIGH-NUTRIENT FOOD CHOICES

- Vitamin B complex providers
  - Beef, whole grains, brown rice, and bran.
- Vitamin C providers
  - Richest source is citrus fruits (orange, grapefruit, lemon, lime, and tangerine).
  - All other fruits and vegetables.
- Vitamin A (beta-carotene) providers
  - All yellow fruits and vegetables.
  - All dark green vegetables.
- Calcium providers
  - Richest source is milk and dairy products (select low-fat and skim-milk products to avoid saturated fat).
  - Canned sardines and salmon, including bones.
  - Dark green, leafy vegetables.
  - Broccoli and rhubarb.
- Protein providers
  - Meat, poultry, and fish.
  - Eggs.
  - Milk and dairy products.
  - Legumes (beans and peas) and nuts.
- Omega-3 fatty acid providers
  - Dark fleshed fish (salmon, tuna, and mackerel), cod, and fish oils.
- High fiber providers
  - Richest sources are cruciferous (cabbage family) vegetables, whole grains, and bran.
  - Cellulose-dense fresh vegetables (carrots and celery) and fresh fruits (eat peels and skins if possible).
- Poor nutrient providers
  - Refined sugar and syrups, refined white flour, and other refined grains stripped of outer coatings.
  - Saturated animal fat and coconut oil and palm oil.
  - Fried foods.
  - Overcooked vegetables.
  - Caffeinated beverages, sweetened drinks, and alcohol.
  - Chemical additives, artificial sweeteners, and flavoring agents found in processed foods.

QUICK GUIDE TO COUNTING CALORIES

Calories do count. Taking in 3,500 excess calories can result in a one-pound weight gain. Taking in 3,500 calories less than you are expending on energy can result in a one-pound weight loss. Just 500 more or fewer calories each day can add up to 3,500 calories in a week—for a one-pound weight gain or loss.

You don't need to count calories fanatically. You can do it in round numbers to get an approximate total and still keep control of how much you are eating in relation to how much energy you are spending. If you can keep these amounts in reasonable balance, you will not add to the fat warehouses of your body, but you will provide adequate nutrients to keep the body in good health.

THE 200 TO 400 CALORIE RANGE

- *Meat.* No matter how you slice it, four ounces of beef amounts to about 300 calories in round numbers. If it is extremely lean beef with all visible fat trimmed away, count it as 250. If it is as fatty as short ribs, count it as 400. Four ounces consists of about two thin slices of meat, one medium-size hamburger, and about half of a sirloin strip steak. Count lean unfried veal as poultry. Count well-trimmed lamb as beef. Count pork as fatty beef.
- *Poultry.* Count four ounces of all poultry as 200 calories, if it has been prepared without any added fat (without butter or frying) and you have not eaten the skin. If it has been prepared in a salad with mayonnaise, add 100 calories for each tablespoon of mayonnaise in your portion. Four ounces is roughly the edible meat of one-quarter of a small chicken. Light meat has less fat and fewer calories than dark meat, but this fast-counting method does not take that into consideration.
- *Fish.* Count 200 calories for four ounces of fish, prepared with no added butter and not fried. Fattier fish such as mackerel has more calories than flounder, but this fast-counting method does not take that into consideration (there is also a positive benefit to the fattier fish: You get omega-3 fatty acids). If you use butter or tartar sauce on the fish, count 100 calories for each tablespoon used.
- *Pies, Cakes, and Cookies.* Figure 300 calories for any serving of fruit pie. Count 200 for plain cake, and 400 for frosted cake. Count two cookies as 200 calories (100 calories each).

THE 100 TO 200 CALORIE RANGE

• *Cheese*. Count all kinds of cheese as 100 calories per serving. A serving is one-half cup of cottage cheese or one ounce of any hard cheese (Swiss, muenster, or cheddar). High-fat and spreadable cheeses (soft cheese such as brie or havarti) count as 125. Use a kitchen scale once to find out what one ounce of cheese looks like, or count a one-inch cube as one ounce. Count one tablespoon of grated Parmesan cheese as 20 calories.

• *Milk*. Count one cup of whole milk as 160 calories. If it's skim milk a cup is only 90 calories. If it's chocolate milk, count one cup as 190. Count one cup of a chocolate milk shake as 350.

• *Ice Cream*. Count one-half cup regular ice cream as 150 calories. If extra rich, count it as 160. If ice milk, count it as 140 calories.

• *Cereals and Grains*. Count all cereals as 100 calories per one-ounce serving. Count all cooked cereals as 100 calories per three-quarter-cup serving. Count one-half cup of cooked rice as 100 calories. Pasta is 210 for each five-ounce cooked serving without sauce; add 30 calories for plain tomato sauce and 150 calories for meat sauce.

THE 0 TO 100 CALORIE RANGE

• *Eggs*. Count 80 calories for each egg that is cooked without butter or other fat (whites are 15 calories each). Add 100 calories for each tablespoon of fat used in the preparation of the egg.

• *Cream*. Whether sweet, whipped, or sour cream, count it as 50 calories per tablespoon. Plain nonfat yogurt counts as only 10 calories per tablespoon.

• *Vegetables*. Count one-half cup of most unbuttered vegetables as 20 calories. Exceptions are cooked dried beans, which count as 80 calories per quarter cup, and potatoes, which count as 90 calories each when baked or boiled and eaten plain. Count coleslaw as 50 calories per one-half cup. Count tomato juice as 20 calories per one-half cup. Eat as much lettuce as you want, but count the dressing at 100 calories per tablespoon.

• *Fruits*. Count apples, pears, and bananas as 100 each. Count grapefruit and oranges as 50 each. Assign 30 calories to each wedge of melon, each peach, one-half cup of unsugared berries, or each slice of raw pineapple. Count orange and grapefruit juice as 50 calories per one-half cup. Figure sweetened canned fruits at 100 calories per one-half-cup serving, unsweetened at 50.

• *Breads.* Count 60 calories for each slice of bread, no matter what kind. Figure rolls and muffins at 150. Count crackers as 25 calories each.

• *Beverages.* Count coffee and tea at 0 calories, unless you add sugar (18 calories for each level teaspoon). Count all sodas as 100 calories for eight ounces, except low-calorie varieties. Count beer as 125 for an eight-ounce glass and hard liquors at 100 calories for one ounce. Count wine at 70 calories for three ounces—double that if it is a sweet dessert wine.

• *Fats and Oils.* Count all butter, margarine, shortening, and oils at 100 calories per level tablespoon. Ditto for mayonnaise, Russian dressing, and tartar sauce.

KEEP MOVING!

How can you burn off excess calories? By incorporating some form of exercise into your daily routine. But the popular exercise saying of "no pain, no gain" is not the way to go. Choose an exercise that is comfortable and enjoyable for you. Try to mix a weightless exercise (such as swimming) with a weight-bearing exercise (such as dancing or walking), so that all of your muscles are called into action and the bone mass of your legs is involved. This prevents your leg bones from becoming brittle, a condition known as osteoporosis.

The chart below lists various types of exercise and the number of calories you burn while doing them. It is followed by the "Muncher's Guide" so you can see how many extra calories you are consuming while "grazing" and how much exercise you will need to burn up those added calories and keep them from becoming added pounds.

QUICK GUIDE TO CALORIES CONSUMED PER HOUR OF EXERCISE

Activity	Gross Energy Cost, Calories Per Hour
Bicycling (5½ mph)	210
Walking (2½ mph)	210
Gardening	220
Canoeing (2½ mph)	230
Golf	250
Lawn Mowing (power mower)	250
Lawn Mowing (hand mower)	270
Bowling	270
Fencing	300
Rowing (2½ mph)	300
Swimming (¼ mph)	300

Walking (3³/₄ mph)	300
Badminton	350
Horseback Riding (trotting)	350
Square Dancing	350
Volleyball	350
Roller Skating	350
Table Tennis	360
Ice Skating (10 mph)	400
Tennis	420
Water Skiing	480
Hill Climbing (100 feet per hour)	490
Skiing (10 mph)	600
Squash and Handball	600
Cycling (13 mph)	660
Scull Rowing (race)	840
Running (10 mph)	900

Source: Statistics from the President's Council on Physical Fitness and Sports, Washington, D.C.

MUNCHER'S GUIDE

Check the chart below for calories, fat, cholesterol, and sodium contents of your favorite snacks and for new snack ideas.

Food	Approximate Amount Per Serving			
	Calories	Fat (g)	Cholesterol (mg)	Sodium (mg)
Breads, Cereals and Other Grain Products				
¹/₂ cup corn chips	70	4	0	108
1 cup popcorn, unsalted, plain	30	trace	0	trace
1 cup popcorn, salted and buttered	50	2	5	213
2 graham cracker squares, plain	60	1	0	86
4 whole wheat crackers, 2 inches square	70	4	0	118
16 cheese crackers, 1 inch square	80	5	10	179
4 saltine crackers, 1⁷/₈ inches square	50	1	4	165
4 round snack crackers, 1⁷/₈ inches in diameter	60	4	0	120
2 breadsticks, unsalted	75	1	1	140
1 slice whole wheat toast	70	1	0	180
Bagel, 3¹/₂ inches in diameter	200	2	0	245

Blueberry muffin, 2½ inches in diameter	135	5	19	198
Bran muffin, 2½ inches in diameter	125	6	24	189
10 thin salted pretzel sticks	10	trace	0	48
⅛ 15-inch cheese pizza	290	9	56	699

Vegetables

½ cup zucchini slices	10	trace	0	2
2 carrot and 2 celery sticks	5	trace	0	10
3 broccoli flowerets	10	trace	0	9
4 cauliflower flowerets	10	trace	0	7
½ cup marinated vegetables, drained	60	5	0	116
½ cup vegetables marinated in no-oil dressing, drained	25	1	trace	75
6 fluid ounces tomato juice	30	trace	0	658
6 fluid ounces tomato juice, no-salt added	30	trace	0	18
1 medium dill pickle	5	trace	0	928
10 potato chips	105	7	0	94
10 salted french fries	160	8	0	108

Fruits

Small apple	60	trace	0	12
¼ cantaloupe	45	trace	0	12
Banana	105	1	0	1
6 fluid ounces orange juice	85	trace	0	2
1 small box raisins, ½ ounce (about ½ tablespoon)	40	trace	0	2
4 dried apricot halves	35	trace	0	1

Milk, Cheese and Yogurt

1 ounce Swiss cheese	105	8	26	74
1 ounce cheddar cheese	115	9	30	176
1 ounce processed American cheese	105	9	27	406
1 cup skim milk	90	1	5	130
1 cup lowfat milk, 2% fat	125	5	18	128
1 cup whole milk	150	8	33	120
8-ounce carton plain lowfat yogurt	145	4	14	159
8-ounce carton lowfat yogurt with fruit	230	2	10	133

Nuts and Seeds

¼ cup salted, roasted peanuts	210	18	0	156
¼ cup unsalted, roasted peanuts	210	18	0	2
¼ cup salted, dry-roasted peanuts	210	18	0	293
2 tablespoons peanut butter	190	16	0	153
¼ cup salted, roasted sunflower seeds	210	20	0	205

Food	Approximate Amount Per Serving			
	Calories	Fat (g)	Cholesterol (mg)	Sodium (mg)

Desserts

Food	Calories	Fat (g)	Cholesterol (mg)	Sodium (mg)
½ cup frozen yogurt	105	2	8	50
½ cup sherbet	135	2	7	44
½ cup ice milk	90	3	9	52
½ cup regular ice cream	135	7	30	58
½ cup chocolate pudding (made with lowfat milk and dry mix)	145	3	9	169
2 chocolate chip cookies, homemade, 2⅓ inches in diameter	90	6	9	41
Frosted brownie, 1½ inches by 1¾ inches by ⅞ inch thick	100	4	14	59
2 chocolate or vanilla sandwich-type cookies	100	4	0	94
2 fig bars	105	2	14	90
2 oatmeal–raisin cookies, 2⅝ inches in diameter	120	5	1	74
Chocolate-frosted cupcake	120	4	19	92
Frosted cream-filled cupcake	160	4	26	194
¹⁄₁₂ 10-inch round angel food cake	125	trace	0	269
⅙ 9-inch apple pie	405	18	0	476
Cake-type doughnut	210	12	20	192
Raised doughnut	235	13	21	222

Food	Approximate Amount Per Serving		
	Calories	Fat (g)	Sugars* (g)

Beverages and Candy

Food	Calories	Fat (g)	Sugars* (g)
12 fluid ounces diet cola soft drink	trace	0	0
12 fluid ounces regular cola soft drink	160	0	39
12 fluid ounces light beer	95	0	2
12 fluid ounces beer	150	0	2
12 fluid ounces wine cooler	175	0	36
1½-ounce chocolate candy bar	220	14	22
10 jelly beans	105	trace	17

*One teaspoon of table sugar equals about 4 g.
Source: USDA Human Nutrition Information Service.

7

FOOD TRICKS THAT KEEP YOU CALM AND HAPPY

A MEAL CAN BE A PLEASANT AND SATISFYing experience, giving visual and gustatory sensations while contributing to feelings of comfort and satiation. But food also plays a biochemical role in the way you function and how you feel. Healthwise, weightwise, and moodwise, it is true—"You are what you eat."

Some people pop pills to regulate their moods. They take downers when they are up and uppers when they are down. Most medications are habit-forming and in due time you will need more and more of them. A better way to control moods is to control your food intake, keeping your blood glucose levels within normal range and avoiding any ingredient that may trigger feelings of depression or fatigue.

Your brain depends on your nutrient intake to function at optimal levels. The brain communicates with the rest of the body by way of neurotransmitters, which "fax" messages between nerve cells called neurons. These instantaneous messages control your movements and your emotions. When you are nutritionally deprived, either or both can go awry.

Your neurotransmitters are "fax ready" only if your diet provides them with the needed nutrients to do their job. Considering that the brain uses 50 percent of the body's supply of fuel (energy) in the form of glucose, the brain will function at the expense of other organs whenever there is a nutrient-poor diet.

Circumstances of malnutrition can become obvious, but borderline subnutrition is more subtle. You may think you are eating well but your food choices may have been stripped of most of their nutritive value before they land on your plate. What isn't on your plate won't be eaten and thus can't be absorbed through your gastrointestinal tract to journey through the blood to a specific site in the brain for conversion by enzymes into neurotransmitters specifically designed to serve particular functions.

Many people seem to be unaware that the human body is so nutrient dependent, particularly on a balanced intake of complex carbohydrates, protein, and fat. The carbohydrates are metabolized into glucose by an intricate series of biochemical steps known as the Krebs Cycle. Vegetable- and fruit-source carbohydrates provide vitamins A and C. Vitamin A is involved in the senses of sight, taste, and smell and vitamin C contributes to the metabolism of carbohydrates into energy-giving glucose. Whole-grain carbohydrates provide the B vitamins, which are vital to memory and brain function.

Carbohydrates need to be a major part of your total food intake each day. Carbohydrates eaten in the form of a simple sugar (sucrose, lactose, honey, or syrup), are swiftly metabolized and can raise your blood sugar level faster than the body can handle it, causing mood swings to occur. The job of insulin, produced by the pancreas, is to control high blood sugar levels. Some people do not produce enough insulin to accomplish this feat—a problem shown at its most extreme as diabetes.

A better way of providing glucose is to increase the complex carbohydrates in your diet, which are converted to glucose more slowly. This prevents a sudden rise and fall of blood sugar and insulin levels. Excess glucose is stored as glycogen. When blood sugar level falls and the body needs energy, a series of hormonal changes takes place, including release of adrenaline, which signals the liver to convert glycogen back into glucose and release it into the system.

The brain is completely dependent on glucose delivered to it via the blood. If the glucose levels in your blood are low, you may feel dizzy and be unable to think clearly. Too much glucose in the blood causes hyper-glycemia (diabetes), while too little causes hypoglycemia. Either condition can wreak havoc with your energy and mood control.

By making a conscious effort to avoid simple sugar (sucrose) and by eating about 68 percent of your daily calories in the form of vegetables, fruits, and whole grains, you will have an adequate storage of glycogen and no jolting blood sugar levels.

Protein provides essential amino acids. These are used as the body's building blocks for repairing tissue and creating neurotransmitters, which send messages from the brain. Protein is also involved in safeguarding the quality of your muscle cells, the connective collagen between your bones, and your hair and nails; protein plays a role in the manufacture of your hormones. While your body can synthesize some of the amino acids it needs, it cannot produce the essential nine that must be in your diet every day. The essential and nonessential amino acids are listed below.

Essential Amino Acids (available only from food)

> Histidine (essential for children)
> Isoleucine
> Leucine
> Lysine

Methionine
Phenylalanine
Threonine
Tryptophan
Valine

Nonessential Amino Acids (synthesized by the adult human body)

Alanine
Arginine
Asparagine
Aspartic Acid
Cysteine
Glutamic Acid
Glutamine
Glycine
Proline
Serine
Tyrosine

Of the essential amino acids, tryptophan is extremely important in brain chemistry. It is involved in regulating mood and sleep and is a precursor to the production of serotonin, a neurotransmitter that affects mood chemistry. Good sources of tryptophan are bananas, beef liver, beef round, lamb, turkey, eggs, almonds, peanuts, and milk.

Methionine, another essential amino acid, can act as an antidepressant when it is combined with vitamin B_{12}. Good sources of methionine plus B_{12} can be found in liver, roast beef, ham, oysters, sardines, herring, milk, eggs, cottage cheese, and yogurt.

Phenylalanine acts with tyrosine as a building block of norepinephrine, a neurotransmitter that stimulates the body to action. Good sources of phenylalanine are eggs, chicken, liver, beef, milk, and soybeans.

Another essential amino acid, lysine, is involved in glucose (energy) metabolism. Good sources of lysine are beef, liver, ham, haddock, turkey, cottage cheese, and milk.

There's no need to run to the corner pharmacy or health-food store to stock up on a supply of amino acids. They are exquisitely proportioned in the protein that you obtain from meat, poultry, fish, eggs, and dairy products. Legumes (beans and peas) also contain good-quality protein, which can be enhanced by eating a grain at the same time. Taking amino acids as supplements should be done only under a physician's close supervision, because this practice could cause an imbalance that would affect your behavior, moods, sleep patterns, and sex drive. Nature has provided you with protein in the right proportions for your needs. Four ounces of lean protein twice a day should be sufficient to keep you calm and your body in good repair. Hypoglycemics seem to need an extra ounce or so of protein between meals—just enough to keep from experiencing hunger pangs.

Research shows that, on average, Americans eat a diet that is composed of a whopping 45 percent fat. Too many people have paid the price with clogged arteries that impede blood flow to the heart and brain, causing heart attacks and strokes. The American Heart Association suggests that no more than 30 percent of our calories should come from fat. Less is even better—except for children who need fat in the diet for normal growth and sexual development.

As people have become more aware of the dangers of a high-fat diet and have learned the difference between saturated and unsaturated fats, the incidence of heart attacks and strokes has been lowered. But a good point to remember is that fat is digested more slowly than carbohydrates and protein. The fat you do eat can be manipulated to keep you calm and in control. For instance, if you have a cracker with cheese before taking an alcoholic beverage, the fat in the cheese will cause the alcohol to stay in your stomach longer, slowing your body's absorption and diluting the effect of the drink. Moreover, it is the fat in your meal that gives you a feeling of satiety. By dividing your daily 20 to 30 percent intake of fat among all of your meals, you will not experience a sluggish reaction to one exceptionally high-fat meal but you will be using your fat intake to stay calm and content.

Eating a wide variety of foods ensures that your body is getting all the necessary minerals as well. Calcium is one of the most important minerals for keeping nerve tissue functioning well. Some calcium absorption can be blocked by eating excess fat and too much oxalic acid (found in spinach and chocolate) and can also be affected by phytic acid found in grains. Although milk and dairy products supply the largest amount of calcium in the diet, good sources are provided by leafy green vegetables, broccoli, sardines, and salmon.

Potassium (found in bananas, strawberries, oranges, and cantaloupe) is involved in transmitting messages between neurons as well as keeping potassium and sodium balanced throughout the body.

Too much sodium can cause fluid retention, which can make you irritable and is related to high blood pressure and kidney problems. If you suffer from PMS, be especially wary of adding salt to food or eating canned soups and processed foods. Fast foods and frozen dinners are especially high in sodium and should be avoided. The irritability and discomfort caused by fluid retention can be overcome by reducing sodium intake throughout the month, and women should especially reduce sodium during the premenstrual part of their cycle.

Minimal amounts of salt are used in the Mood-Control recipes in this book, while herbs and spices are added to give extra flavor. In addition, avoid heavily salted items such as sauerkraut, pickles, processed foods, and deli meats. It is estimated that 2,500 milligrams of sodium a day is enough to keep your cellular balance, and you get that much naturally from the food you eat without adding any salt. Whenever you do add salt to a dish, remember that a level teaspoon of salt contains 2,500 milligrams of sodium. You can readily see that by eating several dishes a day with that amount of added salt, your share will be several times greater than what your body requires. Once you train your taste buds to demand less salt, you will soon discover and enjoy the true flavor of your food while overcoming the dangers of fluid retention.

Chromium is a mineral that plays a role in regulating blood sugar, which in turn is vital for providing energy to the brain. Chromium works together with insulin (produced by the pancreas) to help keep energy (glucose) levels steady. You can guarantee a supply of this important mineral by eating meat, shellfish, chicken, whole grains, corn oil, brewer's yeast, and mushrooms. Avoid the last two if you are sensitive to yeast and fungus.

Green leafy vegetables supply cobalt, a mineral that is an essential part of vitamin B_{12}. Cobalt deficiency may cause thyroid dysfunction, which in turn affects brain chemistry. Excess thyroid hormones can cause irritability and agitation, while a lack of thyroid hormones can cause a debilitating lethargy.

Iodine is the mineral most responsible for thyroid function. A sluggish thyroid gland can cause lethargy, weight gain, and depression. Foods that can block the thyroid's uptake of iodine are called goitrogens—they include cruciferous vegetables (cabbage, broccoli, cauliflower, Brussels sprouts, kohlrabi). Foods that are rich in iodine include fish and iodized salt.

Copper is another important mineral that plays a role in mood control. It assists iron absorption, which in turn produces red blood cells that deliver oxygen to every part of the body. Copper is also needed to make nerve fibers and helps the amino acid tyrosine in its neurotransmitter role. Good sources of copper are almonds, walnuts, avocados, dried prunes, legumes, bananas, mushrooms, oysters, shrimp, and cocoa.

Iron, as stated, is necessary for maintaining a good supply of red blood cells, which are needed by the entire body and certainly by the brain. You can get some of this vital mineral by cooking with old-fashioned cast-iron pots and skillets. Whenever you eat an iron-rich food (organ meats, clams, brewer's yeast, oysters, dried prunes and raisins, eggs, and most beans) try to include foods containing vitamin C in the same meal—this vitamin will increase the body's ability to absorb iron. Try to avoid drinking caffeinated beverages such as coffee, brewed tea, cocoa, and cola drinks when you eat iron-rich foods because caffeine inhibits the absorption of iron.

Magnesium is considered to be an antistress mineral. It is involved in the metabolism of blood sugar into energy. A deficiency of this mineral can cause depression and irritability, while an overdose of magnesium can cause disorders of the nervous system. To stay in calm balance, include the following foods in your diet: bran, brown rice, beef, soybeans, avocados, spinach, and blackstrap molasses.

Manganese is a mineral needed by the enzymes that convert protein into amino acids (some of which are converted into neurotransmitters). It is also involved in the metabolism of glucose and fatty acids. You run little risk of a deficiency of this mineral because it is contained in nuts, whole grains, legumes, and in most vegetables and fruits.

Molybdenum is the cofactor (helper) of several enzymes that are involved in metabolism and the body's iron storage system, but the amounts needed are minuscule and deficiency is unlikely. You get an intake of molybdenum when you eat whole grains, organ meats, legumes, and milk products.

Phosphorous is also involved in metabolism and the transmission of messages in the brain. It is an important part of bone and tooth formation, working with calcium and vitamin D. One reason not to depend on antacids is that this medication tends to destroy phosphorous and can leave you feeling weak. Foods rich in phosphorous include meat, milk, legumes, nuts, seeds, broccoli, and cereal.

Selenium works with vitamin E in the body's antioxidant system, but is only needed in small amounts and it would be rare to have a deficiency. You get selenium whenever you eat bran, tuna, liver, onions, garlic, tomatoes, broccoli, and wheat germ.

We need zinc to optimize our use of vitamin A (needed for night vision) and for communication between brain cells. A deficiency of this mineral can affect your sense of taste and smell, which in turn can affect your appetite. Too much zinc can inhibit the absorption of calcium, and can cause emotional problems and nausea. Good sources of zinc are oysters, beef, lamb, tuna, eggs, whole grains, and cranberries.

You can readily understand why a varied diet is essential if you yearn to be free of food-related mood swings and aim for peace and serenity. Every meal should provide as wide an assortment of nutrients as possible to allow your brain and nervous system to function at their highest level throughout the day.

It is not just what you eat at meals that counts, it is what you reach for midmorning and midafternoon that can affect the way you feel. Why fill up on snacks of nutrient-stripped soda, cookies, or candy that deliver no nutritional benefit or slow burn or energy? Instead of drinking several cups of coffee with doughnuts or Danish pastry between meals, carry along some snacks that have nutritional value; they will actually calm your nerves and focus your thoughts. All are easily packed into sandwich-size plastic bags and most do not have to be refrigerated. They can be tucked into a handbag or attaché case for a calming "munch break."

CALMING MUNCH BREAKS

Unsalted dry-roasted peanuts
Unsalted almonds
Raisins
Cubes of hard cheese
Salt-free peanut butter spread on salt-free wheat crackers
Sugar-free yogurt
Apples
Bananas
Other fruit in season
Unsalted popcorn

For more information about the role of vitamins and minerals, see chapter 9 where supplementation and safety limits are discussed.

Nutrients not only interact with each other but they also interact favorably or unfavorably with medications and other substances that you ingest. Besides eating enough food to satisfy your appetite, consider whether what you are eating is going to do you any good. The next chapter will explain how nutrients interact with other substances and what you can do to make these interactions positive ones.

8

SUBSTANCE ABUSE AND FOOD INTERACTIONS

WE NOW KNOW IF YOU OVERINDULGE IN some substances (tobacco, alcohol, and drugs) you can become dependent on them to feel okay. Often, overindulgence in these substances is caused by a wish to blot out feelings, to suppress depression, or to mask fatigue.

Cigarette smoking is no longer considered sophisticated behavior. The consequences of smoking are serious enough that cigarette packages now carry the statement "Surgeon general's warning: Smoking causes lung cancer, heart disease, emphysema, and may complicate pregnancy." Tobacco companies also use the alternate statement "Surgeon general's warning: Cigarette smoke contains carbon monoxide." People have been alerted to their right to uncontaminated air and smoking-privileged areas have become more clearly defined. Those people who continue to smoke tobacco do so at great risk.

People who consume alcohol and drugs are also at risk. Famous sports figures and film stars have made television ads warning about alcohol and drug abuse and pleading as candidly as possible for you to get help and kick these habits before the habits kick you.

Prescribed medications now come with warning labels about whether to take them before, after, or between meals, because of the possibility of food interactions that may change the effectiveness of the drug. Self-prescribed drugs, both over-the-counter and street drugs, are being used rampantly, without regard to the physical and mental damage that can eventually ensue. As all pharmaceuticals become more sophisticated, consumers must also become more sophisticated about their use and abuse.

When does using a substance such as tobacco, alcohol, or drugs become abuse? When it interacts with and depletes the nutrients you've eaten, rendering them useless; when it does bodily harm; and when you are so hooked on the substance that you can no longer take it or leave it. Being informed is the first step to reasonable action.

TOBACCO/NUTRIENT INTERACTION

Some people use cigarettes as one way to control their weight. While nicotine can increase your metabolic rate to burn food faster, it does so only if you are engaged in some activity. If you are passively smoking while having a coffee break, the nicotine won't speed metabolism. Exercise will speed up your metabolism all by itself!

Those who gain weight when they stop smoking generally do so in the period immediately after they stop. It is possible for nicotine withdrawal to produce a craving for sweets, and the desire to snack is increased by the habit of frequently putting something in your mouth. Be aware of this situation and have low-calorie snacks (fresh fruit, popcorn, celery chunks) or sugarless chewing gum on hand. Also, step up your exercise during the withdrawal period to distract you, prevent weight gain, and help you feel athletic and in control.

Some people smoke cigarettes to have something to do with their hands. What about fingering worry beads, a smooth stone, a crystal segment, a marble, or a coin? If the problem is to relieve tension, there are safer ways to do it than polluting your body.

Some people think smoking is sexy. This myth is perpetuated in old movies and in cigarette ads. But, while those scenes of lighting two cigarettes and swapping passion-filled glances cause excitement on the screen, in real life, they cause yellow teeth, stained fingers, and the lingering odor of tobacco in your hair and on your breath. Not very sexy!

It is generally agreed that you deplete about twenty-five milligrams of vitamin C per cigarette smoked. According to a study by Canada's Bureau of Nutritional Sciences, conducted over a two-year period and covering a cross section of the Canadian population ranging in age from twenty to sixty-four, the vitamin C blood level of smokers who consumed twenty cigarettes or more a day was much lower than that of nonsmokers. This is alarming, because vitamin C is needed for almost every metabolic process of the body.

Free radicals, contained in cigarette smoke, have been linked to arthritis, cancer, lung disease, heart disease, skin aging, and senility. Vitamin C is necessary to prevent these degenerative diseases. If you do smoke, you should be sure to eat foods high in vitamin C (citrus fruits and vegetables) and supplement your vitamin C intake throughout the day. Other vitamins possibly depleted by smoking are vitamins B_{12} and B_6 (found in beef and whole grains), which are needed for brain chemistry (see chapters 7 and 9).

Studies dating as far back as 1939 demonstrate that tobacco smoke can impair the body's processing of proteins and carbohydrates. To add fuel to the fire, cigarette smoke contains an increased amount of toxic trace metals. These metals (cadmium, lead, arsenic, and selenium) can accumulate in the body and cause damage. (Selenium in trace amounts is necessary for health, but in larger quantities it becomes toxic.)

Finally, the Harvard Medical School Health Letter reported a twofold increase in risk for miscarriages and lower birth weights in infants of mothers who smoke, and for women and men alike they reported an increase in facial wrinkling, a decreased sense of smell and taste, the possibility of a constant cough, and an increased danger of injury by fire.

When you smoke cigarettes, you inhale noxious tar and carbon monoxide, along with deadly nitrosamines. This endangers those who are nearby. Most of all, however, smokers interfere with the oxygen delivery system of their own bodies. More than 50,000 scientific studies have shown that smoking is a preventable cause of chronic illness, nutrient depletion, lung disease, and heart disease. In the United States, smoking is responsible for one death in six. If you are a smoker, please consider stopping. Your life may well depend on it.

ALCOHOL/NUTRIENT INTERACTION

If you have an occasional glass of wine about twice a week, or a drink of hard liquor at random social events, you have little risk of significant nutrient depletion as a result of alcohol consumption. But if those social occasions happen daily; if you finish off a bottle of wine with your meal, or if you frequently consume a six-pack of beer in an evening, the risks are great.

Alcohol has a toxic effect on many organs, particularly the liver. A healthy liver can dilute the alcoholic content of a one-half-ounce drink in an hour, preferably on a full stomach. Two dry martinis take the average person four hours for the effects to wear off by oxidation via the bloodstream.

You can consider one drink to be one can of beer, a four-ounce glass of wine, one shot glass (one and one-half ounces) of alcohol straight or on the rocks, or one mixed drink. If you drink on an empty stomach, one drink can have the effect of two or more. That's why cheese and crackers, chips and dips, and other snacks are usually offered with cocktails. Salty snacks should be avoided because they increase thirst and make you drink more. It's wise to have a small meal (a meat, chicken, or fish sandwich) before you attend an event where drinks will be served.

While an alcoholic beverage does provide many calories, it does not provide the protein, fats, vitamins, and minerals necessary for proper metabolic processes. For alcoholics, drinking frequently takes the place of eating. One pint of eighty-six proof alcohol provides about 1,500 empty calories, satiating the appetite without providing essential nutrients.

Besides causing liver damage, alcohol has been shown to have a direct effect on the digestive system, interfering with the absorption of nutrients. Alcoholics often suffer from malnutrition; their blood levels are low in thiamine (vitamin B_1), vitamin A, and folic acid. Vitamin A depletion can cause night blindness. Alcohol also decreases the concentration of the amino acid tryptophan, lack of which has been implicated as a cause of some depressions.

Prolonged drinking can also cause delirium tremens often referred to as the d.t.'s or "the shakes." A person with the d.t.'s hallucinates as a result of nerve damage caused by malnutrition.

While most people consume alcoholic beverages to feel relaxed, they may also be taking medications for the same reason. Alcohol should never be combined with drugs. Alcohol affects the central nervous system and can interact with sleeping pills, antihistamines, narcotic analgesics, and tranquilizers. You could be courting loss of consciousness, a coma, or death when you mix alcohol with any of these drugs!

Pregnant women should avoid all alcoholic beverages. Studies show that alcohol contributes to low birth weight babies and to fetal alcohol syndrome. When drinks are taken while the fetus is forming, physical deformities, brain damage, and retardation can result. Researchers at the University of Missouri-Columbia School of Medicine report that the ingestion of alcohol during pregnancy may affect the developing fetus's ability to later reproduce and have children. The risks are just too great to take a chance on self-gratification when pregnant.

There are about 10 million alcoholics (one of every ten adults) in the United States. An alcoholic is a person who cannot control his or her drinking, resulting in problems that affect job performance and family life. One of the first signs is that the person needs more and more alcohol to achieve a desired mood. Another sign is denial of a drinking problem while continuing to drink more often and in larger amounts. Despite knowing such drinking will have destructive consequences, alcoholics become so accustomed to alcohol that they may suffer from withdrawal symptoms if they don't have a regular supply.

Professional help is needed to detoxify and counsel both the alcoholic and his or her family. Support groups such as Alcoholics Anonymous exist to assist with this problem. It's important to try to help an alcoholic face facts early and get the problem under control. Hundreds of thousands of alcoholics have recovered and stayed sober for the rest of their lives.

For them, alcoholism is an addiction and a disease and must be treated accordingly.

PRESCRIPTION DRUG/NUTRIENT INTERACTION

If you are taking a prescribed medication you should ask your physician and pharmacist about the possible complications and interactions with nutrients as well as with other medications. If you are seeing several different physicians, always take along the names and dosages of all medications you take. This will help you avoid problems that range from inhibiting the absorption of the medication to disturbing the absorption or elimination of important nutrients.

Some prescribed medications are effective precisely because they block specific nutrients. Be careful not to increase your intake of those nutrients when taking the medication, as you may undermine the desired effect.

If a prescription medication is to be taken over a long period of time, there is more probability that a nutrient deficiency might develop unless specific foods containing that depleted nutrient or supplementation of that nutrient is provided. For example, if you took diuretics on a long-term basis, you would risk the possibility of a potassium imbalance. For some people, eating more potassium-rich foods (bananas, oranges, melons, and strawberries) is enough to stay in balance. For others, potassium supplementation should be prescribed. Your physician should be taking blood tests to determine your needs.

Some foods actually enhance absorption of drugs into the bloodstream, while others interfere with it. That is why you should obtain specific directions if you want to get the full benefit from your prescription. Your pharmacist should be able to give you the information you need. Ask whether the medication should be taken on an empty stomach before meals, on a full stomach after meals, or whether there is any food or drink that will interfere with the action of the drug.

A classic example of such interference is that between the antibiotic tetracycline and milk or other dairy products. The calcium in the milk inhibits the absorption of the tetracycline.

Blood-thinning drugs (anticoagulants) do not mix well with foods high in vitamin K, such as liver and green leafy vegetables. Vitamin K is needed for blood clotting, while the anticoagulant is prescribed to prevent blood clotting. These drugs also do not mix with alcoholic beverages.

Monoamine oxidase (MAO) inhibitors, which are prescribed for depression, can interact with the chemical amine tyramine, which is contained in cheese, chicken liver, and red wine. The list of other foods to avoid when taking a MAO-inhibiting medication includes those containing yeast and those that have undergone fermenting processes and aging processes. These foods include pickled herring, yogurt, salami, soy sauce, raisins, bananas, avocados, cola beverages, coffee, chocolate, and alcoholic beverages.

Another group of drugs used to combat depression is tricyclic antidepressants. These should never be combined with alcoholic beverages. Antibiotics, antihistamines, and insulin also should not be combined with alcohol.

Regular use of antacids, whether prescribed or over-the-counter, may cause a deficiency of phosphates, causing muscle weakness and possible vitamin D deficiency. Some antacids contain aluminum hydroxide, which leads to loss of phosphorous, a cause of weak and brittle bones. Aluminum also has a suspected connection with Alzheimer's disease and should be kept out of the diet.

While aspirin is a fairly safe medication, frequent use can cause bleeding of the digestive tract, leading to iron deficiency. Aspirin may cause reduced folic acid levels as well as deplete the vitamin C in the body.

Laxatives may deplete some vitamins. The safest ones to take are those that provide fiber or are in the class of stool softeners. Such old standbys as mineral oil cause loss of the fat-soluble vitamins, A, D, E, and K. Loss of these vitamins disturbs calcium metabolism, which can lead to loss of bone mass, known as osteoporosis. If you eat enough fiber (twenty to thirty grams daily), laxatives should not be needed.

Some commonly prescribed medications and the vitamins and minerals they deplete are listed below. To discover the foods rich in these nutrients, see chapter 9.

Drug or Class of Drugs	Nutrient Affected
Anticonvulsants	Folic acid, vitamins D and K
Anticoagulants	Vitamins A and K
Antihistamines	Vitamin C
Barbiturates	Folic acid; vitamins A, C, and D
Cholestyramine	Folic acid; vitamins A, B_{12}, D, and K
Colchicine	Vitamins A and B_{12}, potassium
Diuretics	Vitamin B complex, potassium, magnesium, zinc
Estrogen contraceptives	Folic acid; vitamins B_1, B_2, B_6, B_{12}, and C

Glutethimide	Folic acid, vitamin D
Indomethacin	Vitamins B_1 and C
Isoniazid	Vitamins B_3 and B_6
Kanamycin	Vitamins B_{12} and K
Neomycin	Vitamins A and B_{12}
Nitrofurantoin	Folic acid
Penicillin	Vitamins B_3, B_6, and K
Phenylbutazone	Folic acid
Prednisone	Vitamins B_6, C, and D; potassium, zinc
Pyrimethamine	Folic acid
Sulfonamides	Folic acid; vitamins B_2 and K
Tetracycline	Vitamin K, calcium, iron, magnesium
Triamterene	Folic acid
Trifluoperazine	Vitamin B_{12}
Trimethoprim	Folic acid

For a more complete understanding of your body's vitamin and mineral needs and how to meet them through your diet, proceed to the next chapter.

9

HOW AND WHEN TO USE SUPPLEMENTS

HOW DO VITAMINS AND MINERALS
KEEP YOU HEALTHY?

CHEMICAL REACTIONS IN THE BODY ARE dependent on the presence of the proper vitamins and minerals, which act as coenzymes to the enzymes manufactured in your body. They are essential helpers that keep your body systems and organs in good working order.

It is rather rare in Western countries to find individuals who have an absolute deficiency of vitamins resulting in one of the easily recognizable vitamin deficiency diseases such as scurvy (a deficiency of vitamin C), or pellagra (a deficiency of vitamin B_3). Unfortunately, it is not rare in our culture to have a depletion of several vitamins, resulting in less than optimum health. Most of the time there is a deficiency in several nutrients at the same time, not just one.

Nutrients may be deficient for a number of reasons, but barring a metabolic disorder (which is certainly not a common cause of deficiency), the most common cause is simply lack of attention to the nutrient intake. People have individual needs for various nutrients. To complicate matters further, each individual's needs change from time to time, depending on other factors such as dietary changes, smoking, use of medication, alcohol consumption, psychological stresses, pregnancy and childbirth, pollution, and physical illnesses.

The tug-of-war between professionals about the pros and cons of taking supplements can sometimes add more confusion then clarity. Advice from respected authorities ranges from "Supplements are unnecessary" to "Everyone can benefit from megadoses of supplements." Who is right? Probably neither extreme is close to the truth.

The common argument from those who advocate that supplements are not necessary is that a well-balanced diet provides all the necessary nutrients and, therefore, supplements are not necessary. True, but how many of us actually eat those theoretical well-balanced meals? And what happens during times of physical and/or emotional stress when our nutritional demands are greater?

Other factors may interfere with obtaining all the necessary nutrients from food even if we do manage to eat a balanced diet. The nutrient content of foods can vary significantly with seasons, with farming techniques, and with the way food is prepared. How many people are aware of when or on which farm their foods are grown? Are most fruits and vegetables eaten raw or slightly steamed to preserve the nutrient content?

One fallacy of arguing that supplements are not needed, is that no wise professor or well-meaning government agency is able to tell you exactly how much of a nutrient is really necessary. The government-issued recommended daily allowance (RDA) is generally accepted as the minimum amount of nutrient advisable to consume daily. This is the level recommended for maintaining life, not necessarily for maintaining optimum health. There is a big difference between the two!

Moreover, the RDA seems to be written in sand. With each new nutritional debate, different recommendations are made. The differences seesaw from year to year. This is why the RDA is not necessarily an infallible guide for nutritional health.

The media often scares us with headlines such as "VITAMINS ARE FOUND TO BE DANGEROUS." The story may relate the effects of overdoses of vitamin A, a fat-soluble stored vitamin that will cause serious problems if taken in large quantities. Some reports will quote studies that prove, for example, that vitamin C destroys vitamin B_{12} or causes kidney stones. Other studies do not come to the same conclusions, but this information never seems to reach the media.

Most of the time, warnings about the danger of taking vitamins really means that there is risk in taking some vitamins in an unsupervised and overzealous manner. The danger is with the improper use of a particular vitamin, rather than a broad implication about the danger of all vitamin supplements. A perfect example of this is the report about several women who sustained neurologic damage after taking relatively large doses of pyridoxine (vitamin B_6) to treat PMS. These unfortunate women demonstrated a point at considerable personal expense. Vitamins may be used in two ways. One way is to ensure proper consumption of nutrients, even if you think you eat well. This extra insurance will compensate for the increased needs your metabolism might demand from time to time, for the lack of any nutrients in the soil your food was grown in, and for the lack of any nutrients in the processed foods you eat. When using supplements for this purpose, large doses of a particular nutrient are usually not needed. The best approach is to take a high-potency multivitamin and multimineral after checking the brand and doses with your doctor. In so doing, you will not be risking a supplement overdose or imbalance and you will be giving yourself some nutritional insurance.

The second way supplements have been used successfully is to treat illness. The women who took vitamin B_6 were attempting to treat an illness, but they didn't have the medical knowledge to realize that the B vitamins are interrelated and that taking large doses of one B vitamin can cause serious deficiencies in other B vitamins.

When supplements are used to treat an illness, professional guidance should be used, as with any treatment of illness. A knowledgeable practitioner would not have prescribed large doses of vitamin B_6 without suggesting the use of other B vitamins and without supervising the patient carefully for side effects.

Finally, it is important to remember that vitamins work together with other nutrients such as minerals, proteins, fats, and carbohydrates. No one has ever been able to sustain life by taking vitamin pills and not eating or by expecting vitamins to supplant the benefits of a nutritious diet. The list below reveals some of the most important functions of particular vitamins and suggests how they may be obtained through diet and a supplement program.

VITAMIN A

- *Deficiency results in:* Dry, rough skin, problems in adjusting to night vision, bright-light sensitivity, tooth decay, and soft tooth enamel.
- *Helps with:* Protecting mucous membranes thus cutting down on colds and sinus infections, may alleviate night blindness, and protects bones and teeth from erosion. Improves dry skin.
- *Found in:* Fish oils (halibut and cod), dairy products, carrots, and green leafy vegetables.
- *Comments:* Too much vitamin A can be dangerous. The toxic level varies for individuals, but it has been claimed that 25,000 IU on a daily basis may be too much for some people. Recently beta-carotene, a very active form of vitamin A, has been made available as a supplement and claims are being made for its benefits. One such claim is that it reduces the rate of lung cancer in smokers to that of nonsmokers. Beta-carotene is also being studied for the protective effect it seems to have from some of the unpleasant side effects of chemotherapy.
- *Caution:* Skin discoloration to an orange hue occurs in people who overconsume carrots or carrot juice in an effort to obtain beta-carotene. If some is good, more may not be!

VITAMIN D

• *Deficiency results in:* Abnormal calcium metabolism, aches and pains of bones, and rickets (the condition of soft bones, resulting in bowed-out leg bones).
• *Helps with:* Prevention of acne, calcium absorption, and bone formation.
• *Found in:* Fish liver oils (cod and halibut are especially good) and dairy products. The body produces its own vitamin D from the action of sunlight on the skin.
• *Comments:* Like vitamin A, vitamin D is a fat-soluble vitamin and is stored in the body. With the possible exception of children under two years of age and pregnant and nursing mothers, 400 IU a day should be sufficient. Most people who are exposed to sunlight need not worry about sufficient vitamin D intake.

VITAMIN E

• *Deficiency results in:* Uncomfortable menstruation, fatigue because of poor oxygenation, poor sperm quality, spontaneous abortions, and poor wound healing.
• *Helps with:* Healing wounds, the body's optimal use of proteins and carbohydrates, and menopausal symptoms. It increases fertility and reduces the incidence of miscarriages.
• *Found in:* Oils such as soy, wheat germ, corn, and peanut; whole grains; eggs; and green leafy vegetables.
• *Comments:* Increasing fertility does not mean that vitamin E acts as an aphrodisiac. Vitamin E is not an aphrodisiac, nor are any of the vitamins. (It is interesting, though, what happens to the sex life of an individual who is experiencing optimum health. Sex, like all body functions, is improved in a healthy person.) The vitamin E found in vegetable oils is easily destroyed by processing. To get the full nutritional benefit from the foods, the oils should be cold pressed. These oils will spoil if left open and not refrigerated, so it is best to buy a small amount of the oil rather than a larger bottle and be sure to store it in the refrigerator. It is also a good idea to buy and use different kinds of oil, because the oils have varying quantities of nutrients. Peanut, soy, corn, and nut oils may be alternated for tasty and nutritious variety.

VITAMIN C

- *Deficiency results in:* Easy bruising and bleeding, especially in the gums; fatigue; poor wound healing; and loss of appetite.
- *Helps with:* Healing wounds and building connective tissue—the mortar of the body. There is a suggestion that vitamin C helps fight toxic chemicals in the body. Some evidence exists for the antiviral effect of vitamin C in large doses. It also has an antihistaminic effect in large doses.
- *Found in:* Citrus fruits, green leafy vegetables, carrots, and onions.
- *Comments:* The body reacts to an overdose of vitamin C with increased gas and diarrhea. Tests have shown that some individuals may need as much as ten times more vitamin C than other people. Other tests have revealed that a person's tolerance for vitamin C may easily double during time of physical stress, such as infection. Some concern has been expressed about the production of kidney stones by large doses of vitamin C. The safest course is to use vitamin C with caution if you are prone to kidney stone formation. Another concern is that vitamin C destroys vitamin B_{12}. The experiment on which this conclusion is based was done in a laboratory in glass dishes, not in humans. When humans who had been taking large amounts of vitamin C were tested for vitamin B_{12} levels, no deficiency was found. Vitamin C is rapidly depleted by smoking and alcoholic intake.

VITAMIN B_1—THIAMINE

- *Deficiency results in:* Memory difficulties, heart rhythm irregularities, leg swelling, irritability, depression, constipation, and lethargy.
- *Helps with:* Circulation, mood, appetite, digestion, and nervous system function.
- *Found in:* Nuts, whole grains, brewer's yeast, and egg yolk.
- *Comments:* Thiamine need frequently increases with heavy alcohol consumption. Thiamine is easily destroyed by high-temperature cooking, boiling in water, and by high-sugar diets.

VITAMIN B_2—RIBOFLAVIN

- *Deficiency results in:* Cracks in the corner of the mouth, light sensitivity, insomnia, fatigue, hair loss, and scaly skin.

- *Helps with:* Integrity of skin around lips, skin texture, and mental alertness.
- *Found in:* Organ meats, milk, and brewer's yeast.
- *Comments:* If you don't eat organ meats, such as liver, it is possible that vitamin B_2 intake will be insufficient. Riboflavin may have to be supplemented because it is not consumed in large quantities in the diets of most people. Whenever taking any of the B vitamins separately it is important to take a B complex as well. The reason for this is that any one of the B vitamins taken in large quantities may cause the loss of other B vitamins through the kidneys.

VITAMIN B_3—NIACIN

- *Deficiency results in:* Nervous disorders including hallucinations, delusions, confusion, diarrhea, skin lesions, fatigue, lack of appetite, and a bright shiny red tongue.
- *Helps with:* Brain and nervous system functioning, reduction of ringing in the ears, and some skin disorders.
- *Found in:* Some beans, whole grains, brewer's yeast, and organ meats.
- *Comments:* Niacin releases histamine, which causes a "flush." After taking niacin as a supplement, a person may look as though the skin has been exposed to the sun for hours without any protection. The reaction may be distressing, but it is not dangerous. If taken in large enough quantities on a regular basis, the flushing doesn't occur. It is important to build up to the larger dosages to avoid a severe reaction. Niacin has been one of the principal vitamins used in the treatment of schizophrenia. It is also known to lower blood lipids, which is why physicians may prescribe it in treating high cholesterol (but this should be undertaken only under your physician's supervision).

VITAMIN B_6—PYRIDOXINE

- *Deficiency results in:* Poor immune response, which makes body more susceptible to disease, and intolerance for carbohydrates.
- *Helps with:* Utilization of carbohydrates, may reduce the pain of menstruation, has helped autistic children, and may reduce the nausea and vomiting of pregnancy.

• *Found in:* Beef liver, blackstrap molasses, whole-grain rice, barley, and corn.
• *Comments:* Don't forget to supplement with other B vitamins when using pyridoxine in large doses.

PANTOTHENIC ACID

• *Deficiency results in:* Fatigue, adrenal exhaustion, poor appetite, sleeplessness, burning sensation on soles of feet, loss of hair color, and a poor immune system.
• *Helps with:* Fighting stress, reduction of burning soles, mood improvement, proper adrenal functioning, and skin health.
• *Found in:* Most vegetables, brewer's yeast, and organ meats.
• *Comments:* Has been found to be of significance in animal life-extension experiments. Other animal experiments have demonstrated deficiency of pantothenic acid may result in duodenal ulcers and increased infections.

CHOLINE

• *Deficiency results in:* Poor functioning of liver, kidneys, and heart.
• *Helps with:* Fat metabolism, proper liver functioning, and memory.
• *Found in:* Organ meats, wheat germ, brewer's yeast, and egg yolk.
• *Comments:* Choline has been used with some success in the treatment of some cases of Alzheimer's disease, a condition of pre-senility.

FOLIC ACID

• *Helps with:* Healthy red blood cells and healthy liver function.
• *Found in:* Dairy products, brewer's yeast, salmon, oysters, chicken, and walnuts.
• *Comments:* Folic acid is also made by bacteria found in the intestines. These bacteria may be destroyed by the use of antibiotics given for the treatment of some infections. Folic acid is destroyed by heat and light.

BIOTIN

• *Deficiency results in:* Sleep disorders and anemia.
• *Helps with:* Proper utilization of fat and protein.
• *Found in:* Brewer's yeast, whole-grain rice, and wheat germ.
• *Comments:* Easily destroyed, like other B vitamins, by heat, exposure to light, and cooking in water.

PARA-AMINOBENZOIC ACID (PABA)

• *Deficiency results in:* Possibly graying of the hair and lack of protection from ultraviolet radiation.
• *Helps with:* Excellent sun screen when applied topically. Reverses and seems to prevent graying of hair in some people.
• *Found in:* Molasses, wheat germ, brewer's yeast, and eggs.
• *Comments:* Nausea may occur in some people who take dosages in excess of 500 milligrams per day. PABA acts as an important stimulant to intestinal bacteria, which produce many B vitamins. These same beneficial bacteria can be destroyed by antibiotics.

VITAMIN B$_{12}$

• *Deficiency results in:* Pernicious anemia, degeneration of nerves, smooth tongue, and fatigue.
• *Helps with:* Proper functioning of the nervous system, elevation of mood and energy, and alleviation of pernicious anemia.
• *Found in:* Brewer's yeast, dairy products, meat, poultry, fish, and eggs.
• *Comments:* Vitamin B$_{12}$ is found only in animal protein or animal products. Strict vegetarians are frequently deficient in this vitamin. In some people, vitamin B$_{12}$ may not be absorbed well by the intestinal tract because of a lack of a substance in the walls of the intestines that is necessary for absorption. In such cases, B$_{12}$ can be supplemented by injections or by the use of a tablet that is absorbed through the veins under the tongue.

MINERALS

Minerals, like vitamins, are necessary for the proper progression of biochemical reactions. Minerals, unlike vitamins, seem to have complicated interrelationships. Some minerals will displace others; some minerals will be retained and used only in the presence of adequate amounts of other minerals. Some minerals are needed in large amounts because of the way they function in the body. Others are needed in trace amounts and may be toxic in large quantities. In other words, be careful with mineral supplementation. The minerals needed in the largest amounts are calcium, magnesium, sodium, potassium, and sulfur.

CALCIUM

- *Deficiency results in:* Irritability, depression, insomnia, pain in the calves, cramps, difficulty in breathing, and bone degeneration (osteoporosis).
- *Too much results in:* Heavy calcification of the bones.
- *Found in:* Dairy products, some beans, hard water, molasses.
- *Comments:* Young children need calcium, as well as good supplies of all nutrients, for proper bone growth. Another group who should watch their calcium intake is postmenopausal women who are susceptible to weakening of the bone structure through excessive calcium loss.

MAGNESIUM

- *Deficiency results in:* Rapid heart beat, twitching, sound sensitivity, depression, and irritability.
- *Too much results in:* Lethargy, stupor, and coma.
- *Found in:* Nuts, whole grains, green vegetables, and seafood.
- *Comments:* Autistic children who were originally treated with large doses of vitamin B_6 and no magnesium were found to be increasingly irritable and experienced bed-wetting. The addition of magnesium stopped those symptoms.

SODIUM

- *Deficiency results in:* Low blood pressure, fatigue, and poor appetite. An acute deficiency, as happens in heat fatigue, may result in serious consequences such as profuse sweating, coldness, stupor, shock, and coma.
- *Too much results in:* High blood pressure, water retention (edema), and irritability.
- *Found in:* Table salt, dried fish, nuts, salted butter, most processed foods such as frozen dinners, canned products, and packaged products.

• *Comments:* Some health conscious people restrict and fear sodium. But sodium is absolutely necessary for life. It is true that most people eat too much sodium, but don't make the mistake of thinking that any sodium is bad. The body's requirement of 2,500 milligrams per day is amply supplied by a diet that includes fresh vegetables and fruits. Processed foods should be avoided. A single item usually contains more salt than anyone needs in one day. A diet heavy in processed foods may supply four times the daily requirement for sodium. Those with kidney problems (which makes it difficult to rid the body of sodium) and those with heart disease and hypertension may need less sodium than the average healthy person. Consult your physician for guidance on your individual sodium requirements.

POTASSIUM

• *Deficiency results in:* Irregular pulse, fatigue, apathy, and muscle cramps.
• *Too much results in:* Poor appetite, muscle fatigue, apathy, and impaired cardiac functioning.
• *Found in:* Whole grains, fruits, potatoes, bananas, and spinach.
• *Comments:* Potassium deficiency, which can result in serious cardiac problems, easily develops in people who take water pills (diuretics) without proper supervision. Diuretics cause a loss of other important minerals, in addition to potassium, and those minerals need to be replaced. Anyone who takes diuretics should have blood tests done on a regular basis to determine mineral levels and should be under the close supervision of a physician.

SULFUR

• *Deficiency results in:* Fatigue.
• *Too much results in:* Toxicity signs not recognized.
• *Found in:* Meat, fish, beans, nuts, eggs, cabbage, and Brussels sprouts.
• *Comments:* Sulfur-containing compounds have been found to act effectively in removing toxic metals from the body, but it is not common to take sulfur compounds as supplements. Beans that have been cooked slowly are a rich natural source of sulfur compounds.

TRACE MINERALS

Minerals that are necessary in small quantities are called the trace minerals. These are lithium, selenium, chromium, manganese, copper, zinc, iron, and rubidium. These are readily available from different foods and are a good reason to eat a varied diet.

LITHIUM

- *Deficiency results in:* Manic-depressive disorder in susceptible individuals.
- *Too much results in:* Tremors, diarrhea, and confusion.
- *Found in:* Mineral waters, whole grains, and seeds.
- *Comments:* The use of lithium for the treatment of manic-depressive illness requires dosages by prescription and with a physician's close supervision. Lithium serum level tests must be done on a regular basis to avoid possible serious toxic effects in manic depressives.

SELENIUM

- *Deficiency results in:* Aging pigment, and increased oxidation.
- *Too much results in:* Fatigue, paralysis, and serious impairment of the nervous system.
- *Found in:* Fish, animal proteins, and whole grains.
- *Comments:* Ongoing studies suggest a possible role for selenium in protecting against the development of some cancers. Until such issues are proven conclusively, however, it is not advisable to self-medicate with selenium supplements.

CHROMIUM

- *Deficiencies result in:* Possible damage to arteries and impaired metabolism of carbohydrates.
- *Too much results in:* No symptoms of toxicity are known.
- *Found in:* Whole grains, brewer's yeast, clams, and liver.
- *Comments:* Chromium helps regulate blood sugar levels and plays a role in diabetes. It is also involved in amino acid metabolism.

MANGANESE

- *Deficiencies result in:* Poor hair and nail growth, loss of hearing, poor muscular coordination, impaired metabolism of carbohydrates, and increased side effects if taking tranquilizers.
- *Too much results in:* Poor appetite and mood and behavioral disorders.
- *Found in:* Whole grains, nuts, and beans.
- *Comments:* Low manganese levels have been found in some people

who suffer from convulsions. Sex hormone production depends on adequate supplies of manganese.

COPPER

- *Deficiencies result in:* Weakness, anemia, breathing problems, and skin sores.
- *Too much results in:* Disorders of thinking, activity, and mood; premenstrual tension; and brittle hair.
- *Found in:* Nuts, shellfish, beans, whole grains, and copper pipes (trace amounts actually enter the water supply).
- *Comments:* Not too many years ago, copper was thought to be harmful to the body. Now it is known that small amounts of copper are needed for proper functioning of many chemical reactions, such as protein metabolism.

ZINC

- *Deficiencies result in:* Loss of taste and smell, prostate problems, impaired growth, hair loss, and white spots on fingernails.
- *Too much results in:* Copper and iron deficiency anemias, nausea and vomiting, and diarrhea.
- *Found in:* Brewer's yeast, seafood, soybeans, whole grains, and mushrooms.
- *Comments:* Semen is rich in zinc. Sexually active men may deplete zinc levels if the diet is not heavy in zinc-rich foods. White spots on fingernails may act as a guide for need for supplementation.

IRON

- *Deficiencies result in:* Anemia, poor concentration, fatigue, depression, and hair loss.
- *Too much results in:* Liver problems, vitamin C deficiency, and iron deposits in body tissues.
- *Found in:* Organ meats, green leafy vegetables, and eggs.
- *Comments:* Iron is stored in the body in healthy people. Unless there is blood loss, adult males rarely need to supplement iron because diet provides sufficient quantities. Menstruating women, on the other hand, experiencing monthly blood loss, may need iron supplementation on a regular basis.

RUBIDIUM

- *Deficiencies result in:* Some work has been underway to investigate the connection between rubidium and depression. The results are not yet known.

- *Too much results in:* Toxic effects are not known.
- *Found in:* Soybeans, muscle meats, milk, and vegetables.
- *Comments:* Rubidium, like other trace minerals, may be necessary to the body in very small amounts, but not enough is known at present to say more. It does serve as a good illustration that we are still discovering new facts about our bodies and the nutrients we need.

We hope that this list of vitamins and minerals will give you some idea of where and how these necessary nutrients function in the body. Too much of any of them may cause as many problems as too little. Bear in mind that the list is not all-inclusive and should be used only as a general guide, not as a bible for nutritional supplementation. Individual vitamins and minerals rarely work effectively to control single symptoms, such as headaches or backaches. Vitamins and minerals work together. It is rare to find a deficiency of just one vitamin or just one mineral. Nature supplies vitamins and minerals together in foods we eat. When using supplements to maintain health, the best practice is follow nature's example and use a multivitamin and multimineral. Taking large doses of a particular vitamin or mineral to treat a disease is sometimes helpful, but should be done only under the advice of a trained medical practitioner. Self-medicating with supplements may have serious consequences.

Because light can destroy the effectiveness of vitamin and mineral supplements, they are generally packaged in dark glass or opaque plastic containers to prevent deterioration. Read the labels on these containers to determine whether fillers were used in the manufacture of the supplements. Whenever possible, select as natural a product as you can find.

However, the best way to ingest nutrients is by eating a varied diet. The Mood-Control Diet that follows will show you how!

10

21-DAY PROGRAM TO CONTROL MOODS

IT MAY BE HARD TO BELIEVE, BUT IN JUST three easy weeks you can learn a delicious way of eating your troubles away. The three weeks of menus that follow are presented in stages, so you can concentrate on eliminating just one or two food categories while replacing them with more favorable choices, depending on your needs as you determined them in chapters 1 through 6. This removes the difficulty patients often find when trying to adhere to a prescribed diet. You will be continuing to eat familiar foods at all times, while learning how to select your meals to provide you with satisfaction, level moods, and high energy.

For instance, the first week you will concentrate only on detoxifying from sugar and caffeine while learning how to increase the amount of complex carbohydrates you eat. Simple sugars, such as refined white sugar, syrups, and the sugars listed on the labels of many manufactured products (they generally end with an "ose": sucrose, glucose, galactose, fructose, maltose, dextrose, and lactose) are all quickly metabolized and absorbed into the bloodstream. This can send moods soaring for a while but within a few hours they will plummet into the pits (see chapter 3 for more information on insulin response). Because simple sugar is not only delivered to your body in the form of refined table sugar but also in most manufactured food products, it is imperative to read labels carefully—the producer of the product will often hide the sugar content by lumping it into the category of "carbohydrates." In reality there is a big difference between our body's use of simple and complex carbohydrates. Complex carbohydrates are metabolized more slowly and feed glucose into the blood in a steadier fashion, preventing a yo-yo of energy and moods.

There's something else you should know about complex carbohydrates. They deliver most of the important vitamins you need every day. That's why nutritionists currently recommend that you have two to four servings of fruit and three to five servings of vegetables per day. In addition, it is recommended that you eat six to eleven servings of grains daily, preferably whole grains.

It's preferable to eat fresh fruit rather than juice so none of the fruit's valuable fiber content is discarded. People watching their sugar intake and limiting the amount of fruit ingested should be especially wary of drinking juice—it takes a lot more fruit to make juice. While fruit contains fructose, which is not as quickly metabolized as refined sugar, it is more quickly absorbed than other complex carbohydrates found in vegetables and whole grains. (For further information, see "What Counts As a Serving," later in this chapter.)

It's wise to have a dark green or yellow vegetable each day to get beta-carotene (a form of vitamin A) and several servings of other vegetables and fruits to obtain vitamin C. Whenever you select a cruciferous vegetable (cabbage, broccoli, Brussels sprouts, kohlrabi, and cauliflower) you help to prevent colon cancer, besides obtaining important vitamins and minerals.

Don't overlook serving legumes several times a week, either in the form of bean soup, split pea soup, or cooked beans. Legumes play a double role in nutrition. They are, of course, a complex carbohydrate, but they also contain nature's most complete vegetable protein. The protein content is lacking a bit in methionine, an essential amino acid, but when legumes are served with a bit of meat or combined with a grain at the same meal, it enhances the protein content. Legumes are also rich in thiamin (vitamin B_1) and pyridoxine (vitamin B_6), as well as iron, calcium, phosphorus, and potassium. In addition, their fiber plays an important role in maintaining a healthy digestive tract.

Caffeine is considered by most people to be a pick-me-up. In actuality it is a downer. It is also an addictive drug with no nutritive value. Properly brewed tea has almost the same amount of caffeine as coffee, but you can reduce that by dunking a tea bag only briefly in boiling water or using fewer tea leaves per cup or pot. Your best bet, however, is to find several herbal teas that you like and use them for a hot beverage whenever you wish.

BETTER MOODS AND TASTY FOODS, WEEK BY WEEK

The Mood-Control Diet offers a step-by-step method for revising your eating habits without making a drastic change all at once. The menu plan of week 1 gives you a good blueprint of the best way to combine protein, fat, and complex carbohydrates. The primary goal of week 1 is to detoxify yourself from refined sugar and caffeine while increasing your intake of complex carbohydrates in the form of more vegetables, fruits, and whole grains for a steady supply of energy to your body. Concentrate on eliminating sugar that week. Don't add it to your beverages or foods. Instead of cookies, cakes, sweet desserts, ice cream, or sherbet, choose unsweetened fresh fruit. At the same time, kick the caffeine habit. Give up coffee, brewed tea, and cola drinks. By the end of the third week, you will have your nutritional act together in three easy stages. Remember that the sole object of week 1 is to detox from sugar and caffeine. Don't worry about other nutrition issues at that time.

By week 2 you will be ready to detox from eating excess protein. You may believe that there's no such thing as excess when it comes to protein, but your body can function very well on as little as eight ounces of protein a day. Most people eat much more than that. This means that you may be taking in more protein at the expense of not getting enough vegetables, fruits, and grains (complex carbohydrates).

Spend week 2 continuing to avoid sugar and caffeine, but concentrate on limiting your protein intake, as directed, so that your body will have a better amino acid balance and be able to synthesize all the proteins it needs. Your hunger will be satisfied by an increase in complex carbohydrates. The objective of week 2 is to learn how to limit servings of protein to the actual needs of your body. Hypoglycemics will be advised to eat an extra ounce of protein between meals to stay off the glucose roller coaster.

It is in week 3 that you will take the greatest nutritional step: learning to detox from excess fat, bringing it to 20 to 30 percent of your total caloric intake, and concentrating on increasing your intake of fiber. Excess fat is implicated in both heart disease and cancer.

Statistics show that most people take in more than 40 percent of their calories in fat. Fat is consumed not only in butter, margarine, and oil, but it also is grained throughout fatty cuts of meat and under poultry skin. Fat is hidden in manufactured products as well, making it imperative to read labels and analyze the content of the food you eat.

Fiber is the food ingredient implicated as being most likely to prevent bowel cancer. Fiber is the nonabsorbable cellulose of vegetables, legumes, fruits, nuts, seeds, and whole grains. While it does not contribute nutrients, the fiber portion of the foods from plant sources continues on through the intestine and eventually bulks up the colon for a faster transit time of the waste products of the body. A diet that is high in refined grains and low in plant fiber can cause a deficiency in some vitamins and minerals, as well as slow down the colon's evacuation process. This not only makes you feel sluggish, it sets you up for disease in later life, because waste material becomes toxic when left too long in the body.

It is thought that the average American daily diet contains only about ten grams of dietary fiber. According to the National Cancer Institute, that figure should be twenty to thirty grams of fiber daily. Too much fiber, however, can rush food through your system and prevent the absorption of trace minerals such as iron, magnesium, and zinc. There is an art to eating a variety of foods to prevent this from happening. See appendix 3 to familiarize yourself with the amounts of fiber provided by different foods.

By the end of the three-week Mood-Control menu plan, you will understand how to control your moods and well-being and you will have the nutritional know-how to do it deliciously and sensibly. You will notice that each menu has "modification" instructions for those who have hypoglycemia, food sensitivities, or yeast infections. Other food-related problems requiring special handling are listed in chapter 20. This is a quick-reference chart listing many other special problems that can be alleviated by careful food choices.

Notice also that each recipe in part II has a subtitle to indicate whether it is dairy-free, egg-free, gluten-free, sugar-free, or yeast-free. If it's possible to tailor the recipe to your needs by adding or omitting an ingredient, the introduction to the recipe will inform you of that, too.

The menus are designed to give you maximum freedom of choice, whether you plan to cook at home or dine at a restaurant. It's important to be able to make wise food selections no matter where you are or what you are doing.

Be aware that many foods (besides legumes mentioned earlier) fit into several categories. Milk, for instance, is a protein. But milk (especially if it is whole milk) also contains fat. Skim milk is your best all-round option. Milk is also an excellent source of calcium. Most bottled milk has vitamin D added to it. Our only other source of vitamin D is sunshine.

You can eat lean beef for its vitamin B complex content as well as for its valuable supply of protein and iron. However, by choosing lean cuts of beef, you can lower the amount of animal (or saturated) fat in your diet.

When you choose a fat, you also have a decision to make. Saturated fat (animal-based fat such as that marbled in and around meat, butter, cream, cheese, and eggs) contributes to high cholesterol levels in the blood. Whenever you select corn oil margarine (unsaturated fat) or vegetable oil such as corn oil, olive oil, sesame oil, and safflower oil instead of a saturated fat, you are practicing better nutrition. The exceptions to this are the vegetable oils palm oil and coconut oil—read the labels of manufactured food products to avoid them whenever possible. It's important to know that all fat, whether saturated or unsaturated, whether butter or margarine, has about 100 calories per tablespoon.

It's best to eat a variety of complex carbohydrates rather than to load up on one plateful of spinach because each vegetable, fruit, and grain has an abundance of a specific vitamin and/or mineral that, taken together, works to advantage in the body. By eating a variety of them every day, you have all bases covered.

One easy way to remember to eat many different foods is by color. If you are facing a colorful assortment of foods on your plate, chances are that you are eating better than if it were all monochromatic. Brown (whole grains), green (vegetables), yellow and red (fruit and vegetables), and white (pasta and potatoes), provide you with a wonderful array of nutrients. In addition, you will want to check to be sure that there are protein, complex carbohydrates, and a little fat on your plate.

BECOMING A GOOD-FOOD DETECTIVE

Here's a quick reference chart to help you to become a good-food detective.

Protein

> Meat (beef, veal, lamb, and pork)
> Poultry (chicken, rock Cornish game hen, duck, and turkey)
> Fish (flounder, haddock, halibut, cod, salmon, red snapper, shrimp, herring, clams, mussels, lobster, etc.)
> Eggs (scrambled, omelets, hard-boiled, soft-boiled, in quiche, in baked goods, etc.)
> Dairy (whole milk, skim milk, buttermilk, cheese, yogurt, sour cream, light cream, etc.)

Simple Carbohydrates

> Sugar (white or brown sugar, corn syrup, maple syrup, any other syrup, honey, or any ingredient with an "ose" ending)

Complex Carbohydrates

> Vegetables of every variety
> Fruits and berries of every variety
> Grains (wheat, rye, barley, oats, rice, buckwheat, millet, etc.)

Fat

> Butter, margarine, shortening, olive oil, corn oil, safflower oil, sesame seed oil, any other oil
> Saturated fat includes any fat from an animal source, including the fat in dairy products
> Polyunsaturated fat includes any fat from a vegetable source, except palm and coconut oils, which have a higher saturation ratio

Monounsaturated fat includes any fish oil, olive oil, and canola oil, which can help lower blood cholesterol levels if taken in reasonable amounts

Sources of Vitamins in Food

Vitamin A (beta-carotene) is found in yellow and dark green vegetables and fruits (broccoli, spinach, turnip greens, acorn squash, carrots, cantaloupe, melon, and apricots)

Vitamin B complex is found in beef and in whole grains (brown rice, wheat bran, oat bran, and buckwheat groats)

Vitamin C is found in high amounts in citrus fruits (orange, grapefruit, lemon, and tangerine) and also in all fruits and vegetables, including those containing vitamin A

Vitamin D is obtained from sunlight and is added to milk

Vitamin E is found in all fats, including fish oils

Armed with this information, you can now look at a plate of food and detect what's in it for you! Where's the protein? Where are the complex carbohydrates? Is there a dark green or yellow vegetable to provide vitamin A's beta-carotene—or have you had a yellow fruit? Have you had a cruciferous vegetable today? Have you had a whole-grain cereal or bread? How about a serving of lean beef to provide vitamin B complex? Is there any unwanted sugar? Is there any unwanted fat? It's a balancing act that can provide you with a safety net of protection and well-being.

In addition, if you are sensitive to major food ingredients such as wheat or milk, you will have to determine whether that is hidden in the food on your plate. Yeast-free dieters will assess the bread and baked goods for yeast content, the salad dressing for vinegar content, and the cheese for mold content, and will also look for mushrooms. You learned in chapter 5 that yeast-free dieters must control sugar intake, so be sure to evaluate sweets and fruits for that purpose. Hypoglycemics and those who love junk food will assess the amount of hidden fat and sugar in the offering. The more fat, sugar, and junk (ingredients and additives without nutritive value) you can get off your plate, the more you can fill it up with high-density nutrients that will help you to feel full and feel well.

Now you are ready to start the Mood-Control Diet! Here is an at-a-glance breakdown of the program:

Week 1: Detox from sugar
Detox from caffeine

Increase complex carbohydrates (fruit, vegetables, and grains)

Week 2: Detox from excess protein

Week 3: Detox from excess fat

Week 3 becomes your maintenance diet. It contains all the nutritional guidelines necessary for optimal health while also helping you eliminate food-related mood problems. Read on, and discover a new way of eating and a new YOU!

MOOD CONTROL WEEK 1: DETOX FROM SUGAR AND CAFFEINE

• Avoid sugar completely. It lurks in alcoholic and other beverages; in desserts such as cakes, cookies, ice cream, and sherbet; and in manufactured canned, packaged, and frozen food products.

• Avoid caffeine. It is in coffee, tea, chocolate, cocoa, and cola drinks. Instead, use decaffeinated coffee and decaffeinated and herbal tea.

• Increase portions of fruits, vegetables, and grains. Aim to eat two to four servings of fruit (hypoglycemia and yeast-free dieters are limited to two fruits a day) and three to five servings of vegetables daily. Aim to eat six to eleven servings of grains daily.

–Have at least one dark green or yellow fruit or vegetable daily

–Have one cruciferous (cabbage family) vegetable daily

–Serve cooked dried beans and peas several times a week, as vegetable, soup, or main entrée

–Choose cooked whole grains (such as brown rice or whole-grain rice instead of refined white rice, kasha, millet, and couscous), whole-grain bread, whole wheat pasta, and whole-grain cold or cooked cereals (such as oatmeal, bran cereal, and shredded wheat) instead of refined cereals

WHAT COUNTS AS A SERVING?

Fruits

• 1 whole fruit such as a medium apple, banana, peach, plum, nectarine, tangerine, or orange

- ½ grapefruit
- 3-inch wedge of melon
- ½ cup any berries
- ½ cup cooked fruit
- ½ cup fruit juice
- ¼ cup dried fruit

Vegetables

- ½ cup cooked vegetables
- ½ cup chopped raw vegetables
- 1 cup of leafy raw vegetables, such as lettuce or spinach

Grains

- 1 slice bread
- ½ hamburger bun or large roll
- 1 small roll or muffin
- 4 small or 2 large crackers
- ½ cup cooked whole grain cereal, no sugar, no additives
- 1 ounce cold whole-grain cereal, no sugar, no additives
- ½ cup cooked whole-grain rice, millet, or kasha
- ½ cup cooked pasta

WEEK 1 MENU PLAN (NO LIMIT ON AMOUNTS)

Breakfast

> Any unsweetened fresh fruit
> Hot or cold whole-grain unsweetened cereal with milk, or
> Eggs, any way
> Toast with any unsweetened topping
> Decaffeinated beverage, herbal tea

Lunch

> Vegetable soup or bean soup
> Sandwich on whole-grain bread, including any poultry, meat, or
>   fish filling as desired, with lettuce and tomato
> Coleslaw
> Decaffeinated beverage, herbal tea

Snack

Fresh fruit, such as banana, apple, pear, etc.

Dinner

Mixed green salad, dressing as desired
Any poultry, meat, or fish, as desired
Baked potato, pasta, brown rice, kasha, or other
    cooked grain
Spinach or carrots, or any dark green or yellow
    vegetable
Berries, unsweetened fruit, or low-sugar cookie
Decaffeinated beverage, herbal tea

Snack

Skim milk with rice cake, plain popcorn, fruit, or
    whatever sugar-free and caffeine-free food desired

Food-sensitivity modification—avoid your trigger food(s), or if tolerable, rotate such food every four days. *Yeast modification*—limit fruit to two servings a day. Avoid bread made with yeast, avoid cakes because of possible yeast and sugar content, avoid alcoholic beverages, vinegar, soy sauce, mushrooms, and moldy cheese (Roquefort, blue, etc.). *Hypoglycemic modification*—limit fruit to two servings a day. Eat protein (milk, yogurt, cheese, peanuts, meat, etc.) between meals.

MOOD CONTROL WEEK 2: DETOX FROM EXCESS PROTEIN

• Limit protein intake to one egg for breakfast if desired and four-ounce servings of poultry, meat, and fish for lunch and dinner. (Four ounces is about the size of a hamburger patty.)
• Count one egg, one-half cup cooked beans, or two tablespoons of sugar-free peanut butter as one ounce of meat.
• The limited protein will allow for more helpings of vegetables and whole grains as patterned in week 1.
• Continue to eat fruits as patterned in week 1.
• Continue to avoid sugar and caffeine.

WEEK 2 MENU PLAN

Breakfast

> Any unsweetened fresh fruit
> Hot or cold whole-grain unsweetened cereal with milk, or
> 1 egg, any way
> Toast with any unsweetened topping
> Decaffeinated beverage, herbal tea

Lunch

> Vegetable soup or bean soup or salad (any dressing)
> Pasta with plain tomato sauce
> 4-ounce serving of poultry, meat, or fish on plate or sandwich
> Any raw or cooked green vegetable
> Decaffeinated beverage, herbal tea

Snack

> Fresh fruit, such as banana, apple, pear, etc.

Dinner

> Any raw vegetable salad with any dressing
> Any 4-ounce portion poultry, meat, or fish
> Any potato, pasta, brown rice, kasha, or other cooked grain
> 1 green cruciferous vegetable (cabbage, broccoli, Brussels
>   sprouts, etc.)
> 1 yellow vegetable (carrots, acorn squash)
> Whole-grain bread as desired
> Berries, unsweetened fruit, or low-sugar cookies
> Decaffeinated beverage, herbal tea

Snack

> Skim milk with rice cake, plain popcorn, fruit, or whatever
>   sugar-free and caffeine-free food desired

Food-sensitivity modification—avoid your trigger food(s), or if tolerable, rotate such food every four days. *Yeast modification*—limit fruit to two servings a day. Avoid bread made with yeast, avoid cakes because of possible yeast and sugar content, avoid alcoholic beverages, vinegar, soy sauce, mushrooms, and moldy cheese (Roquefort, blue, etc.). *Hypoglycemic modification*—limit fruit to two servings a day. Eat protein (milk, yogurt, cheese, peanuts, meat, etc.) between meals.

MOOD CONTROL WEEK 3: DETOX FROM FAT

• Limit use of butter, margarine, and shortening. Each tablespoon of fat contains 100 calories. When reading labels, remember that each gram of fat has 9 calories, as opposed to 4 calories each for protein and carbohydrates.

• Limit use of mayonnaise, sour cream, all other creams, creamy salad dressings, and whole-milk products, and use skim milk, nonfat yogurt, and low-fat cheese instead.

• Limit egg yolks to only two or three per week. There's no limit on egg whites except to count it as pure protein.

• Use only lean cuts of meat, trimming all visible fat before eating. Remove skin from poultry and discard—fat lurks beneath that skin, especially on duck. Dark meat is fattier than light meat, so try to consume more light meat.

• Continue all the modifications you practiced in week 1 and week 2. Avoid sugar and caffeine. Continue to have at least two to four servings of fruit, three to five servings of vegetables (including one dark green or yellow vegetable and one cruciferous vegetable) daily. Continue to use whole grains instead of refined grains whenever possible.

• Aim to have 20 to 30 percent of your daily calories as fat. Try to consume most of it in the form of unsaturated vegetable oil whenever possible. Whenever you have an egg yolk or eat other extra animal fat, take care to restrict other fats in that meal or on that day.

WEEK 3 MENU PLAN

Breakfast

>Any unsweetened fresh fruit
Hot or cold unsweetened whole-grain cereal with skim milk, or
1 egg (only 2 or 3 times a week), scrambled in a nonstick skillet, poached, or boiled
Whole-grain toast with any unsweetened topping, such as low-

fat cottage cheese or dietetic jelly
Decaffeinated beverage, herbal tea

Lunch

Vegetable soup or bean soup (no creamed soup), or salad with
low-fat dressing (buttermilk, vinegar and oil in limited
amount, lemon juice, or prepared low-fat product)

Any pasta, potato, brown rice, kasha, or other cooked grain
without added fat

Any 4-ounce portion of poultry, meat or fish, not fried, no fat
added—poached, broiled, braised or baked—on plate or
sandwich

Any raw or cooked green vegetable

Decaffeinated beverage, herbal tea, or skim milk

Snack

Fresh fruit, such as banana, apple, pear, etc.

Dinner

Any raw vegetable salad with low-fat dressing as listed for lunch

Any 4-ounce portion of poultry, meat or fish, not fried, no fat
added—poached, broiled, braised or baked

Any pasta, potato, or brown rice, kasha or cooked grain with no
added fat

One green cruciferous vegetable (cabbage, broccoli, Brussels
sprouts, etc.), no butter or fat added

One yellow vegetable (carrots, acorn squash), no butter or fat
added

Whole-grain bread as desired

Berries, unsweetened fruit, or 2 low-sugar cookies

Decaffeinated beverage, herbal tea, skim milk

Snack

Skim milk with rice cake, plain popcorn, fruit, or whatever
sugar-free and caffeine-free food desired

Food-sensitivity modification—avoid your trigger food(s), or if tolerable,
rotate such food every four days. *Yeast modification*—limit fruit to two

servings a day. Avoid bread made with yeast, avoid cakes because of possible yeast and sugar content, avoid alcoholic beverages, vinegar, soy sauce, mushrooms, and moldy cheese (Roquefort, blue, etc.). *Hypoglycemic modification*—limit fruit to two servings a day. Eat protein (milk, yogurt, cheese, peanuts, meat, etc.) between meals.

Remember that week 3 becomes your maintenance menu. Using it, along with your knowledge of your own body's special nutrient needs, you can now dine in any restaurant and know how to order the healthiest available food. Eating at home gives you even more freedom: total control over freshness, health-smart ingredients, and food-safety practices. The cooking advice and recipes in part two will help you to enjoy delicious meals while regaining your energy and zest for living.

PART TWO

THE MOOD-CONTROL RECIPE SECTION

CHOOSING FOOD WISELY

WHETHER COOKING AT HOME OR ORDER-
ing in a restaurant, the Mood-Control Diet is easy to follow. You make the
choices. There is plenty of leeway for your personal preferences. Here's
what you need to know.

When dining out, scan the menu for food that can be cooked to order.
Ask specific questions about the way the dish you order will be prepared.
Give the waiter instructions if there are ingredients that should be omitted.
Try to order food selections that are broiled, baked, or steamed. Breaded,
fried foods are taboo. Have your salad brought with dressing on the side, so
you can control the amount you use. When helping yourself to a salad bar,
choose the fresh and simple vegetables—avoid the mayonnaise-loaded
offerings. Use the salad dressing ladle with care—you could be choosing a
healthful salad and pouring a 400-calorie ladleful of fat on your food.

Restaurant cooks often make use of the same overprocessed high-
additive dehydrated and processed food products that you've been cau-
tioned to omit at home. Frozen portion-controlled food and microwave
ovens can really fool you if you don't know the food business. A visit to a
national hotel and restaurant supply convention is a rude awakening to the
fact that fresh food may not be on the menu, unless you are in a notable
chef's domain.

To get the best nutrient delivery, when studying a menu, ask yourself
whether you are ordering simple fresh food. Broiled fish or chicken, a baked
potato, steamed spinach, and a green salad would be the way to go. Fresh
berries, melon, or fresh fruit cup are wise dessert choices.

At home, you have more control over your nutrient intake. The recipes
in the Mood-Control Recipe Section have been deftly devised to give you
delicious meals. All are easy to prepare. Note that the recipes are all low in
fat and cholesterol, low in sodium, and free of refined white sugar and
white flour.

Eggs are used as a source of protein in some main entrée dishes. It is
recommended that you eat only one egg at a time, and limit eggs to two or
three a week, if your blood cholesterol level is higher than 200. Nutritionists recommend that you limit yourself to 300 mg of cholesterol a day. Using

our recipes, it's easy to know whether you are doing that. Every recipe has been analyzed for nutritional content and calories. That information appears at the bottom of each recipe, so you can make knowledgeable choices.

Sometimes there is no time to cook after a busy day. You will find a section of recipes that do not require any cooking but deliver a punch of nutrients anyway. Other evenings when you in a hurry but want a hot meal, use a recipe that advises you of short cooking time. There are many of them in the "Easy Entrée" chapter.

Think pasta when you are in a rush—it cooks in twelve minutes while you prepare a sauce. Some pasta recipes take more time, such as the baked lasagna combinations. They can be made in advance and reheated quickly.

Soups have been included for moments when you want the pleasure of such sustenance. It's a good way to add beans, lentils, and vegetables to your meal. If there are leftovers, freeze them for another day. Canned soups are very high in sodium and the low-sodium varieties taste awful to most people. Better to make your own, stocking a variety of soups in your freezer.

The selection of vegetable recipes should spur you to enjoy the flavor and texture of these wonderful vitamin and mineral providers. Buy vegetables in small amounts that you can use within a few days, keeping every serving fresh, fresh, fresh!

Experiment with plain steamed or boiled grains, such as kasha (buckwheat groats), millet, barley, wild rice, and brown rice. Bake a sweet potato or yam for beta-carotene content. Learn to enjoy a baked white potato without adding butter, margarine, or sour cream—use plain low-fat yogurt on it if you must.

Dessert should be a piece of fresh fruit. The dessert chapter in this book can be used for those once-in-a-while occasions when a little fussing is desired.

FOOD SAFETY AND HEALTH PRECAUTIONS

If you have a healthy respect for the safety precautions that should be observed when handling food, you'll be able to avoid the nation's leading food hazard: food poisoning due to bacterial growth. The symptoms of such illness include nausea, diarrhea, and stomach cramps—sometimes all at once. The way to prevent food poisoning is to be aware that it is caused by faulty food-handling practices, in your own home or in other homes and restaurants.

Some bacteria are harmless and others are actually helpful when they stay where they belong, but they become harmful when outside their normal surroundings. A combination of such bacteria exists in the gastrointestinal tract. Unwashed hands between bathroom and kitchen can spread harmful bacteria to your food. In addition, bacteria that exist on the skin, nose, and in the throat can be transmitted to food by touch, sneeze, or cough. There's no sense in becoming a hypochondriac about it, fearing food contamination, but there is sense in washing your hands often and preparing your meals under the cleanest of conditions.

In addition, there are organisms that normally exist on food, some of which can be destroyed by refrigeration, freezing, and proper cooking techniques. You should know about them. The forms of bacteria that can cause food poisoning are *Salmonella, Staphylococcus, Clostridium perfringens,* and *Clostridium botulinum.* The latter is rare but can be fatal.

Some households seem to have a situation where a "virus" is always attacking its members. Often that "virus" is mishandling of food. Here are the precautions you should learn to practice to avoid bouts of food poisoning in your life.

Salmonella organisms may be found on raw animal products, such as meat, poultry, and eggs. (This is one good reason never to buy cracked eggs and always to rinse off the eggshells before breaking them open.) Refrigeration and freezing will retard the growth of salmonella, so it's most important that these products be transported from market to refrigerator with all due speed. Cooking destroys this bacteria. If you eat dishes such as steak tartare that are made with raw ground beef, you are at risk!

Some bad kitchen habits can also unwittingly place you at risk. When handling a chicken, rinse first, then keep it on the paper or plastic bag it came in, or lay out a fresh sheet of wax paper on which to work. Then after the chicken is in the pot or pan, gather up the mess and toss it in the trash. Never place your chicken on a counter and then prepare fresh salad greens in the same spot! The greens will pick up any bacteria on the raw chicken and you'll be playing health-hazard roulette. If you don't use this preventive measure, at least wash the counter with soapy water and rinse thoroughly before bringing on the greens. Once the chicken is cooked, the problem no longer exists.

When *Staphylococcus aureus* organisms, which abound on the skin, in the hair, in the nose, and in the throat, are transmitted to food, they multiply quickly at room temperature and form a toxin. Unfortunately, cooking does not necessarily destroy this toxin. Food that is left at room temperature after being infected with this toxin and then reheated will be a possible source of food poisoning.

Watch out for food preparers with a cold, a cough, or open skin sores. If that someone is you, be careful about using clean utensils to mix the food and keep the golden rule of the kitchen: Keep food hot (above 140° F) or cold (below 40° F) and above all, keep food clean.

Clostridium perfringens are organisms that occur in soil and in the gastrointestinal tract of humans and animals. Spores (the inactive forms of bacteria) may be on raw meat and poultry and can be activated if left at room temperature even after cooking. Only refrigeration can hold this bacteria in check. So if you roast a chicken ahead of time, don't let it stand in the kitchen for hours until dinner is to be served. Refrigerate it as soon as possible (yes, even when still hot) and reheat just before serving.

The last and most vicious bacteria is *Clostridium botulism*, which is found in soil and in water. Improper canning practices are the major cause of this organism getting into the food supply. A simple precaution is never buy a can of food that has a bulging top, and when you use a can you have stored for a while discard it if there is any evidence of rust, leaking, or bulging top. Don't taste it; this type of food poisoning really can be deadly!

"Waste not, want not," may be a good rule to follow when planning purchases, but, "when in doubt, throw it out," has its place in food practices as well. Here are some other rules to observe to prevent bouts of food poisoning:

- Always purchase perishables last.
- Always get perishables home fast.
- Always buy foods from below the frostline in your store's freezer cabinet; the ones on top may have been thawed and refrozen several times.
- Keep meat and poultry in the refrigerator up to three to five days; otherwise, store in airtight wrappings in the freezer.
- Never keep food at room temperature longer than two hours, and preferably less; observe this rule when serving a large crowd and keep backup portions in the refrigerator rather than setting it all out, if the party is to last many hours.
- Refrigerate leftovers in tightly covered containers as soon as possible after serving; when reheating, cook thoroughly.
- Stuff poultry just before roasting and remove stuffing to refrigerate separately.
- Don't touch your nose, mouth, or hair when preparing food; wash hands frequently and avoid using hands on food; and when it's necessary to knead dough be most careful.
- Throw food out if you suspect that it has a chance of being contaminated; you will not be able to see, smell, or taste the contamination!

- Observe the kitchen golden rule: Keep food hot (above 140° F) or cold (below 40° F) and above all, keep food clean—use extreme caution with food at room temperature.

QUICK GUIDE TO THE NUTRITIONAL ANALYSES

All recipes are followed by a computer analysis based on data from the U.S. Department of Agriculture's (USDA) *Composition of Foods*. Recipes are not only marked with calories per portion, but also with nutrient content expressed in grams or milligrams.

- Total calories for the day should be composed of
  12 percent of calories in protein
  20 to 30 percent of calories from fat
  58 to 68 percent from carbohydrates
- Convert grams of protein and carbohydrates into calories by multiplying the number of grams by four (10 g × 4 = 40 calories).
- Convert grams of fat into calories by multiplying the number of grams by nine (10 g x 9 = 90 calories).
- Total the number of calories you eat each day and then break it down into the total number of calories eaten as protein, carbohydrates, and fat to determine whether you are patterning the percentages of protein, carbohydrates, and fat, as listed above.
- Cholesterol intake should be no more than 300 milligrams per day.
- The National Cancer Institute recommends twenty to thirty grams of fiber per day, but no more than thirty-five grams (see appendix 3 for a list of the fiber content of foods).
- Sensible sodium intake should be about 2,500 milligrams per day (see appendix 4 for a guide to the sodium content of foods).
- Aim for 1,000 to 1,200 milligrams of calcium a day.
- Women and teenagers should aim for eighteen milligrams of iron a day and men should have ten milligrams of iron a day.
- Potassium intake has a wide range for adults, 1,875 to 5,625 milligrams of potassium should do the trick.

11

HEALTHIER SNACKS AND APPETIZERS

We have all lived through decades of dips and chips that add up to an overload of fat and sodium. But the comparison chart on the facing page shows how we pay the piper health-wise when we choose chips over fresh vegetables. It has become accepted fare for convivial party goers, but it is possible to adapt low-fat offerings with crudités (crisp raw vegetables) and present a more healthful party platter. You will find several low-fat dips in this chapter.

There are also spreads that have had the fat deftly removed, leaving it up to you to serve with an assortment of whole-grain crackers or Scandinavian crisp bread. Or go the Tex-Mex route and offer salsa as an alternative spread. It is available in jars or you can make your own with just a little effort.

When just grazing for snacks at home, be sure to have an air popper to make your own fresh unbuttered, unsalted popcorn. Sprinkle with garlic powder or onion powder to get a heightened flavor.

Unsalted peanuts mixed with raisins makes another healthful snack. Toss in some crunchy spoon-size shredded wheat cereal to the mixture. Select low-sodium, low-fat cheese for a better punch of protein and calcium. Stuff celery hollows with low-fat cottage cheese and enjoy a crunchy moment.

Use these recipes as party fare, a first course, or a snack. It's smart to nibble the healthier way!

VEGETABLES OR NACHOS

Vegetables = Raw vegetable platter (carrots, zucchini sticks, and cherry tomatoes)
Nachos = Twelve tortilla chips with one-quarter cup cheese sauce
  Calories
   Vegetables = 30
   Nachos = 285
  Fat (g)
   Vegetables = 0
   Nachos = 19
  Sodium (mg)
   Vegetables = 15
   Nachos = 965

Source: USDA Human Nutrition Information Services.

FRUIT JUICE SWIZZLER

(dairy-free, egg-free, gluten-free, sugar-free, yeast-free)   *Makes 1 serving*

If you think that you drink too many soft drinks, taking in excess sugar calories or chemicals (in the case of sugar substitutes found in diet sodas), here's a neat way to cut down and still have a fizzling beverage.

INGREDIENTS
4 ounces any fruit juice
4 ounces club soda or seltzer
Mint sprig for garnish

Just before serving, stir liquids together and pour over ice cubes in a glass. Garnish with mint sprig.

NUTRITION PER SERVING

		Calories:	55		
Carbohydrate:	13 g	Cholesterol:	0 mg	Potassium:	248 mg
Protein:	1 g	Fiber:	.1 g	Calcium:	14 mg
Total Fat:	0 g	Sodium:	1 mg	Iron:	.3 mg

AVOCADO YOGURT DIP

(egg-free, gluten-free, sugar-free, yeast-free)   *Makes 1 cup*

Avocados take kindly to yogurt in this zesty dip. Be sure to add the lemon juice to keep the avocado from turning brown.

INGREDIENTS
1 very ripe avocado
1 drop Tabasco sauce
¼ teaspoon salt
2 teaspoons lemon juice
1 tablespoon prepared white horseradish
½ cup plain nonfat yogurt

Peel avocado and remove pit. In a medium bowl, mash avocado well. Add Tabasco sauce. Stir in salt, lemon juice, horseradish, and yogurt. Mix well and chill for at least 1 hour. Serve as a dip for vegetables, fresh fruit slices, or crackers.

NUTRITION PER TABLESPOON

		Calories:	27		
Carbohydrate:	1 g	Cholesterol:	.1 mg	Potassium:	100 mg
Protein:	.7 g	Fiber:	.2 g	Calcium:	16 mg
Total Fat:	2 g	Sodium:	34 mg	Iron:	.08 mg

CRUDITÉS AND DILLED DIP

(egg-free, gluten-free, sugar-free, yeast-free)   *Makes 8 servings*

Raw vegetables marry well with a zippy-flavored low-fat dip. Here's a way to get your vitamin A with ease.

INGREDIENTS
2 carrots, scraped, cut into 3-inch sticks
2 cups broccoli flowerets
1 cup cauliflower flowerets
1 cup plain nonfat yogurt
½ teaspoon dried dill
½ teaspoon prepared white horseradish
1 tablespoon grated Parmesan cheese

Arrange vegetables on a platter. Crisp in the refrigerator until ready to serve. For a dip, combine yogurt, dill, horseradish, and Parmesan cheese in a medium bowl. To serve place bowl in the center of the vegetable platter.

NUTRITION PER SERVING (½ CUP)

		Calories:	39		
Carbohydrate:	6 g	Cholesterol:	1 mg	Potassium:	270 mg
Protein:	4 g	Fiber:	.9 g	Calcium:	111 mg
Total Fat:	.2 g	Sodium:	18 mg	Iron:	.5 mg

SALSA FRESCA

(dairy-free, egg-free, gluten-free, sugar-free)   *Makes 1³/₄ cups*

When it comes to salsa, some like it hot and some like it not so hot. This version is fairly mild—add extra jalepeños, if desired. Serve as a dip with taco bits or whole-grain crackers. Yeast-free dieters may substitute lemon juice for the vinegar.

INGREDIENTS
1 cup finely chopped fresh tomato
½ cup finely chopped onion
¼ cup finely chopped coriander leaves
1 teaspoon vinegar
1 small jalepeño pepper, may be canned

Combine tomato, onion, coriander, and vinegar in a small bowl. Remove seeds and membrane from the jalepeño and chop very fine. Add to the tomato mixture. Cover and let stand at room temperature about 5 hours before serving.

NUTRITION PER TABLESPOON

		Calories:	3		
Carbohydrate:	.7 g	Cholesterol:	0 mg	Potassium:	31 mg
Protein:	.14 g	Fiber:	.09 g	Calcium:	3 mg
Total Fat:	0 g	Sodium:	1 mg	Iron:	.09 mg

HERBED YOGURT CHEESE SPREAD

(egg-free, gluten-free, sugar-free, yeast-free)   *Makes about 1 cup*

You can make your own soft low-fat cheese from yogurt. Just mix as directed in the recipe and suspend over a bowl until a soft creamy cheese forms. You'll love it!

INGREDIENTS
2 cups plain nonfat yogurt
1/2 teaspoon garlic powder
1/2 teaspoon dried tarragon
1/2 teaspoon dried dill

In a medium bowl stir all the ingredients together quickly; do not break down the thick consistency of the yogurt. Pour into a large cheesecloth-lined fine-mesh strainer, suspended over a bowl or pot. Let drip at room temperature for about 6 hours. What remains is a soft creamy herb cheese spread. The whey (liquid) is highly nutritious and may be added to soup.

NUTRITION PER TABLESPOON

		Calories:	16		
Carbohydrate:	2 g	Cholesterol	.5 mg	Potassium	72 mg
Protein:	1.6 g	Fiber	0 g	Calcium	56 mg
Total Fat:	trace	Sodium:	7 mg	Iron:	.02 mg

TUNA-CHEESE SPREAD

(egg-free, gluten-free, sugar-free)   *Makes 1 1/2 cups*

Tuna is a good source of Omega-3 fatty acids. A bit of white horseradish gives a tang to this recipe.

INGREDIENTS
1 (7-ounce) can water-packed tuna, drained and flaked
1/4 cup low-fat cottage cheese
4 tablespoons plain nonfat yogurt
2 tablespoons grated onion
1 teaspoon prepared white horseradish
1 teaspoon capers (optional)
1/4 teaspoon Worcestershire sauce

Mix tuna and cottage cheese together in a medium bowl. Add yogurt, onion, horseradish, capers, and Worcestershire. Mix well. Chill.

NUTRITION PER TABLESPOON

				Calories:	14		
Carbohydrate:	.3 g	Cholesterol:	.2 mg	Potassium:	32 mg
Protein:	3 g	Fiber:	trace	Calcium:	8 mg
Total Fat:	.08 g	Sodium:	3 mg	Iron:	.1 mg

BELGIAN ENDIVES AND CAVIAR

(gluten-free, sugar-free, yeast-free)   *Makes 20 hors d'oeuvres*

Here's the way to make one special vegetable such as Belgian endive form the base for a popular appetizer. Dipped or stuffed, the endive leaves make wonderful finger food and are low in calories.

INGREDIENTS
2 Belgian endives
¼ cup low-fat cottage cheese
¼ cup plain nonfat yogurt
1 teaspoon lemon juice
1 hard-cooked egg
1 (2-ounce) jar red lumpfish eggs (caviar)
Fresh dill to garnish

Run cold water over Belgian endives and pat them dry. Separate the leaves, choosing about 20 medium-size leaves. (Save the others for a salad.) Mix cottage cheese, yogurt, lemon juice, and egg into a smooth paste, using an electric blender or food processor, if desired. Place a heaping teaspoon of the mixture in the center of each endive leaf. Top with a dab of caviar. Sprinkle with dill. Arrange on a serving dish in a circle with the tips toward the rim of the dish, to form a pattern like the spokes of a wheel. Refrigerate until ready to serve.

NUTRITION PER SERVING (EACH STUFFED LEAF)

				Calories:	15		
Carbohydrate:	.4 g	Cholesterol:	14 mg	Potassium:	26 mg
Protein:	1.5 g	Fiber:	.02 g	Calcium:	19 mg
Total Fat:	.7 g	Sodium:	66 mg	Iron:	.4 mg

PICKLED SHRIMP

(dairy-free, egg-free, gluten-free, sugar-free) Makes 10 servings as an hors d'oeuvre

*Here's an easy way to serve shrimp for a party. Be sure to have wooden picks
and paper napkins available for comfortable handling.*

INGREDIENTS
1½ pounds shrimp (about 30 medium shrimp)
2 onions, thinly sliced
5 bay leaves
2 tablespoons corn oil
¼ cup water
½ cup tarragon vinegar
½ teaspoon salt
2 teaspoons celery seed
Dash of Tabasco sauce

Rinse shrimp and place in a medium pot, covered with water. Bring to a
boil, cover, and simmer over low heat for 5 minutes. Drain and remove
shells. Devein by removing dark residue along the back of each shrimp.
Rinse again and arrange in a small flat container. Add onions and bay leaves.
Combine oil, water, vinegar, salt, celery seed, and Tabasco sauce; pour over
shrimp. Cover tightly and marinate in the refrigerator for several hours or
overnight. Serve cold as a pick-up appetizer.

NUTRITION PER 3-SHRIMP SERVING

		Calories:	71		
Carbohydrate:	2 g	Cholesterol:	66 mg	Potassium:	134 mg
Protein:	9 g	Fiber:	.07 g	Calcium:	35 mg
Total Fat:	3 g	Sodium:	174 mg	Iron:	.9 mg

CHOPPED CHICKEN LIVERS WITH SHERRY

(dairy-free, gluten-free, sugar-free)   *Makes 1½ cups*

*If you are tired of paying high prices for small portions of chopped chicken liver,
it's time to learn how easy it is to make your own. Yours will be healthier as well,
because the livers will be simmered in liquid rather than fried. Yeast-free dieters
should omit the sherry.*

INGREDIENTS
1 pound fresh chicken livers
1 onion, thinly sliced into rings
1 hard-cooked egg
$1/4$ teaspoon salt
$1/8$ teaspoon pepper
1 tablespoon dry sherry

Wash chicken livers and cut away any green areas. Be sure that the gall sac is not attached (it's dark green in color). Place chicken livers and onion rings in a large skillet. Barely cover the bottom of the skillet with water. Cover and simmer for 5 minutes, turning the livers occasionally and adding a little more water if needed to keep livers from sticking to the pan. Chop or grind the livers, onions, and hard-cooked egg together; stir in just enough pan juices to hold the mixture firmly together. Add sherry. Chill until ready to use.

NUTRITION PER TABLESPOON

		Calories:	37		
Carbohydrate:	.9 g	Cholesterol:	68 mg	Potassium:	36 mg
Protein:	5 g	Fiber:	.01 g	Calcium:	4 mg
Total Fat:	1 g	Sodium:	36 mg	Iron:	1.6 mg

PIZZA ON PITA ROUNDS

(egg-free, sugar-free)   *Makes 2 servings*

Who doesn't like a pizza snack once in a while? You can buy mozzarella cheese that is made from part skim milk to lower your fat intake, and still enjoy the pleasure of a last minute snack that is mighty good!

INGREDIENTS
1 pita bread (round Middle Eastern bread)
4 tablespoons canned tomato sauce
2 teaspoons oregano
4 slices mozzarella cheese, diced
2 tablespoons grated Parmesan cheese

Open pita bread into 2 round pieces. Arrange pita rounds on a cookie sheet, crust side down. Spread each with 2 tablespoons tomato sauce. Sprinkle with oregano. Top with diced mozzarella cheese. Sprinkle with grated Parmesan cheese. Bake in a 350° F oven for 15 minutes, or until cheese is melted.

NUTRITION PER SERVING

		Calories:	246		
Carbohydrate:	8 g	Cholesterol:	49 mg	Potassium:	128 mg
Protein:	16 g	Fiber:	.6 g	Calcium:	423 mg
Total Fat:	16 g	Sodium:	141 mg	Iron:	.7 mg

12

BETTER BREAKFASTS

TRY NEVER TO SKIP BREAKFAST. IT IS A good energy start to the day. Just be sure that the fuel you use to rev up your engine is highly nutritious. Complex carbohydrates in the form of grains and fruit are a good choice.

There's nothing better for you than a bowl of cereal. Be sure it is a whole grain with no added sugar or additives. Best bets are hot cooked oatmeal, Wheatena, or cold cereals such as shredded wheat or bran flakes, without additives. Use skim milk and add some sliced bananas or other fruit to add extra nutrients to the meal.

If your blood cholesterol level is normal, there's no reason why you can't have an egg twice a week. Boil it, scramble it in a nonstick skillet, or make an omelet out of it. Just don't fry it, and certainly don't serve it with bacon. If cholesterol is a problem, consider making an omelet with just the egg whites. The trick is to lightly beat the whites until they are frothy, then add some finely diced onion and parsley and cook in a nonstick skillet.

The traveler's breakfast of pancakes dripping with syrup and melted butter is a horror story. But there's no reason not to have the pancakes—in fact, you'll find several wholesome pancake recipes in this chapter. But they are all cooked on a nonstick griddle and served with applesauce or berries. It's the way to go!

GRANOLA MUNCH

(*dairy-free, egg-free, yeast-free*)   *Makes 14 ¹/₂-cup servings*

Make your own granola to eat as a crunchy-munchy snack or with milk as a breakfast food. Either way, it has less sweetener and more nutrition than manufactured products. Some gluten-free dieters are also sensitive to oats.

INGREDIENTS
3 cups uncooked old-fashioned oat cereal
1¹/₂ cups wheat germ
¹/₂ cup chopped almonds
¹/₂ cup sesame seed
¹/₄ cup hulled sunflower seed
¹/₄ cup honey
1 cup seedless raisins

Combine all the ingredients except the raisins in a large bowl and mix well. Spread the mixture evenly in a nonstick 9 × 13-inch baking pan. Bake in a 300° F oven for 30 minutes, stirring occasionally until lightly toasted. Stir in raisins. Cool. Refrigerate, covered.

NUTRITION PER SERVING

		Calories:	190		
Carbohydrate:	25 g	Cholesterol:	0 mg	Potassium:	274 mg
Protein:	7 g	Fiber:	.6 g	Calcium:	36 mg
Total Fat:	8 g	Sodium:	116 mg	Iron:	.4 mg

HERBED CHEESE OMELET

(*gluten-free, sugar-free, yeast-free*)   *Makes 2 servings*

It is always wise to have eggs in the refrigerator. They can be used at any meal as an omelet and, with varied fillings, can be counted on for good protein and trace mineral nutrients. Fat for cooking can be eliminated if you use a nonstick skillet.

INGREDIENTS
2 eggs
¹/₈ teaspoon salt
2 teaspoons cold water
2 ounces low-fat cheese, diced
1 teaspoon fresh or dried chives

In a small bowl beat eggs lightly, add salt and water, and beat again. Pour egg mixture into a nonstick skillet over medium heat. As the egg solidifies, push it gently toward the center of the skillet, allowing the liquid egg to flow to the edges and solidify. Sprinkle cheese on one-half of the omelet. When the surface is almost dry, flip the other half of the omelet over the cheese and slip the omelet onto a plate. Cut in half and sprinkle with chives.

NUTRITION PER SERVING

Calories: 96

Carbohydrate:	2 g	Cholesterol:	275 mg	Potassium:	89 mg
Protein:	15 g	Fiber:	0 g	Calcium:	46 mg
Total Fat:	6 g	Sodium:	194 mg	Iron:	1 mg

SCRAMBLED EGGS PROVENÇALE

(dairy-free, gluten-free, sugar-free) *Makes 4 servings*

Eggs are the answer to an almost empty refrigerator dinner. As long as you have a few of them and some herbs on the shelf, you'll be able to beat up a fanciful repast.

INGREDIENTS

4 eggs

1 teaspoon prepared mustard

1 teaspoon parsley

1/4 teaspoon salt

1/8 teaspoon pepper

2 scallions, thinly sliced

1 ripe tomato, peeled and chopped

1 tablespoon corn oil margarine

In a medium bowl beat together eggs, mustard, parsley, salt, and pepper. In a large skillet cook scallions and tomato in margarine for about 4 minutes over medium heat, or until vegetables are tender. Add egg mixture and scramble to desired consistency.

NUTRITION PER SERVING

Calories: 108

Carbohydrate:	3 g	Cholesterol:	274 mg	Potassium:	150 mg
Protein:	80 g	Fiber:	.2 g	Calcium:	36 mg
Total Fat:	9 g	Sodium:	245 mg	Iron:	1.2 mg

BLUEBERRY PANCAKES

(*yeast-free*)   *Makes 16 pancakes*

Make your own pancakes this no-yolk low-cholesterol way. Yeast-free dieters should omit the honey.

INGREDIENTS
2 cups unbleached flour
¼ cup nonfat dry milk
2 teaspoons baking powder
1½ cups water
¼ cup corn oil
1 teaspoon honey
2 egg whites
½ cup fresh blueberries

Combine flour, dry milk, and baking powder in a large bowl. Add water, corn oil, and honey; mix together. In a medium bowl beat egg whites until stiff peaks form; fold into batter. Add blueberries. Pour ¼ cup of the batter onto a hot nonstick griddle. Pour as many more batches of batter as will fit. Cook over medium heat until bubbles form and bottoms are lightly browned. Turn and cook on other side until browned.

NUTRITION PER PANCAKE

		Calories:	97		
Carbohydrate:	14 g	Cholesterol:	.2 mg	Potassium:	43 mg
Protein:	2 g	Fiber:	.1 g	Calcium:	24 mg
Total Fat:	3.6 g	Sodium:	53 mg	Iron:	.5 mg

OATMEAL-RAISIN PANCAKES

(*sugar-free, yeast-free*)   *Makes 4 servings*

Here's a way to have your oatmeal disguised as pancakes. Serve with unsweetened applesauce topping, if desired. Some gluten-free dieters are not affected by oats.

INGREDIENTS
1 egg
¾ cup skim milk
1 teaspoon frozen apple juice concentrate

1 cup quick-cooking rolled oats
1½ teaspoons baking powder
¼ cup raisins

In a medium bowl beat egg. Add milk and apple juice concentrate. Add oats and baking powder. Add raisins. If batter is too thick, add a little more milk. Drop by spoonfuls onto a hot nonstick skillet and cook until lightly browned on one side. Turn and brown the other side.

NUTRITION PER SERVING

		Calories:	97		
Carbohydrate:	16 g	Cholesterol:	69 mg	Potassium:	204 mg
Protein:	6 g	Fiber:	.2 g	Calcium:	97 mg
Total Fat:	2 g	Sodium:	296 mg	Iron:	1 mg

LEMON YOGURT PANCAKES

(sugar-free, yeast-free)   *Makes 4 servings*

Use lemon yogurt for extra flavor in these breakfast pancakes. Check the label to be sure the yogurt is sugar-free. Top with puréed fresh berries, if desired.

INGREDIENTS
1 cup unbleached flour
1 teaspoon baking powder
½ teaspoon baking soda
1 egg
1 cup skim milk
½ cup lemon low-fat yogurt

Combine flour, baking powder, and baking soda in a medium bowl. In a small bowl beat egg lightly and add milk; stir into flour mixture. Stir in yogurt. Drop by spoonfuls onto a hot nonstick skillet. Brown on one side, then turn and brown other side.

NUTRITION PER SERVING

		Calories:	170		
Carbohydrate:	29 g	Cholesterol:	70 mg	Potassium:	221 mg
Protein:	10 g	Fiber:	.1 g	Calcium:	158 mg
Total Fat:	1.7 g	Sodium:	130 mg	Iron:	1.2 mg

FRENCH TOAST

(*sugar-free*)   *Makes 4 servings*

When you're down to your last egg and a few not-too-fresh slices of bread, you can combine both into a tasty meal. A helpful trick to know when there's not much to round up in the refrigerator!

INGREDIENTS
1 egg
1/2 cup skim milk
1/2 teaspoon vanilla extract
4 slices day-old whole wheat bread
1/4 teaspoon cinnamon

In a small pan beat egg. Add milk and vanilla; beat well. Dip bread into batter, soaking it in on both sides. In a nonstick skillet over medium heat, brown bread on one side, then turn and brown on the other. Sprinkle with cinnamon.

NUTRITION PER SLICE OF TOAST

		Calories:	94		
Carbohydrate:	14 g	Cholesterol:	69 mg	Potassium:	95 mg
Protein:	6 g	Fiber:	2.1 g	Calcium:	33 mg
Total Fat:	2 g	Sodium:	145 mg	Iron:	.9 mg

HOT RICE AND PINEAPPLE

(*dairy-free, egg-free, gluten-free, yeast-free*)   *Makes 4 servings*

This makes a delicious breakfast dish that can be served as a side dish with chicken or turkey, if desired. The honey may be omitted.

INGREDIENTS
2 cups hot cooked brown rice
2 tablespoons dried raisins
1/4 cup unsweetened pineapple tidbits, drained
1 teaspoon honey
1/8 teaspoon cinnamon
Dash of nutmeg

Combine rice, raisins, pineapple, honey, cinnamon, and nutmeg in a medium bowl. Toss well with a fork. Spoon into cereal dishes.

NUTRITION PER SERVING

		Calories:	145		
Carbohydrate:	32 g	Cholesterol:	0 mg	Potassium:	131 mg
Protein:	2.5 g	Fiber:	2.6 g	Calcium:	18 mg
Total Fat:	.5 g	Sodium:	276 mg	Iron:	.7 mg

13

SATISFYING SOUPS

$\mathcal{S}$OUP IS A COMFORT FOOD. THE LIQUID contains many nutrients that are leached out during cooking. When soup is homemade, you can be certain of the ingredients—for example, the sodium content, which is frequently high in processed products. Homemade soup can last in the refrigerator for up to a week and in a freezer for months.

Old-fashioned cooks started with a basic vegetable-and-bean soup, adding leftover vegetables and pasta to it to change its flavor daily. By practicing "refrigerator roundup" you can do that, too.

The only restriction to making soup is time and imagination. Water is the basic ingredient of most soups. The rest is vegetables; dried legumes; barley, rice, or pasta; and seasonings to balance the flavor. Turn a plain vegetable soup into a tomato soup by adding a can of tomato paste. For a change of pace one day, purée the portion in a blender or food processor. Then heat up the thickened soup, top with popcorn or croutons, and serve.

Use your food processor to make fresh gazpacho as well. All you need is a surplus of tomatoes and a token of other vegetables, with garlic as the kicker seasoning.

If you are a working person, the best time to make soup is on the weekend. Cook it low and slow. Soup has a hospitality all its own!

QUICK VEGETABLE BISQUE

(egg-free, gluten-free, sugar-free, yeast-free)   *Makes 2 servings*

You can make a quick "creamed" soup from any leftover cooked vegetable and then season it with appropriate herbs. If a thicker soup is desired, add a few tablespoons of nonfat dry milk.

INGREDIENTS
1 cup cooked vegetables (broccoli, spinach, carrots, etc.)
1 cup skim milk
1 teaspoon cornstarch

¼ teaspoon salt
⅛ teaspoon pepper
⅛ teaspoon dried dill

Combine all the ingredients together in an electric blender or food processor. Purée. Cook in a small pot, over low heat, stirring constantly, and serve.

NUTRITION PER SERVING

		Calories:	68		
Carbohydrate:	10 g	Cholesterol:	2 mg	Potassium:	410 mg
Protein:	7 g	Fiber:	1 g	Calcium:	221 mg
Total Fat:	trace	Sodium:	338 mg	Iron:	.6 mg

GAZPACHO

(dairy-free, egg-free, gluten-free, sugar-free)   *Makes 4 servings*

When fresh tomatoes are plentiful, here's a way to turn them into a refreshing cold soup. Yeast-free dieters may substitute 1 tablespoon lemon juice for the vinegar.

INGREDIENTS
4 large tomatoes, quartered
1 small onion
1 cucumber, peeled and sliced
1 green pepper, quartered
2 garlic cloves
2 tablespoons wine vinegar
1 tablespoon olive oil
½ teaspoon salt
¼ teaspoon pepper

Purée all the ingredients together in an electric blender or food processor. Pour into a large bowl and chill.

NUTRITION PER SERVING

		Calories:	77		
Carbohydrate:	12 g	Cholesterol:	0 mg	Potassium:	435 mg
Protein:	2 g	Fiber:	1.4 g	Calcium:	35 mg
Total Fat:	3 g	Sodium:	12 mg	Iron:	1 mg

BEAN SOUP

(dairy-free, egg-free, gluten-free, sugar-free, yeast-free)   *Makes 10 servings*

Cook this on the weekend and coast all week. Beans are an alternate source of protein and fiber.

INGREDIENTS
1 cup great northern dried beans
2 quarts water
1 onion, finely diced
2 carrots, scraped, sliced, finely diced
2 celery stalks, finely sliced
2 parsnips, scraped, finely diced
1 turnip, peeled, finely diced
2 garlic cloves, minced
1 dill sprig
1 parsley sprig
1 teaspoon dried basil
1/2 teaspoon salt
1/4 teaspoon pepper

Soak the beans for 1 hour in water to cover in a large soup pot. Pour off the water and add the remaining ingredients. Cover with 2 quarts of water. Cover and cook over low heat for 3 hours, or until beans are tender. Stir occasionally.

NUTRITION PER SERVING

		Calories:	78		
Carbohydrate:	17 g	Cholesterol:	0 mg	Potassium:	261 mg
Protein:	3 g	Fiber:	3.3 g	Calcium:	35 mg
Total Fat:	.3 g	Sodium:	109 mg	Iron:	1 mg

WHITE BEAN SOUP

(dairy-free, egg-free, gluten-free, sugar-free, yeast-free)   *Makes 8 servings*

If you soak the beans in water for several hours or overnight, they will be easier to cook. This is the kind of hearty soup that can become a meal in itself when served with warm bread and a salad. If there will be no other protein in the meal, add cooked rice to each bowl. When combined, legumes and grains supply the essential amino acids found in the protein of meat, poultry, fish, and eggs.

INGREDIENTS
2½ cups dried white beans
1 quart water
2 tablespoons olive oil
1 garlic clove, minced
1 onion, finely chopped
1 carrot, scraped and finely chopped
1 stalk celery, finely chopped
1 ham bone
½ teaspoon dried rosemary
½ teaspoon salt
¼ teaspoon pepper

Soak the beans overnight in 1 quart of water in a large bowl. Heat olive oil in the bottom of a large soup pot. Sauté garlic, onion, carrot, and celery over medium heat until lightly browned. Add beans, including the soaking water. Add ham bone, rosemary, salt, and pepper. Add an additional quart of water. Simmer gently (low heat) for 2 hours, or until beans are tender. Remove ham bone. Rub half the beans through a sieve and stir them back into the soup.

NUTRITION PER SERVING

		Calories:	103		
Carbohydrate:	14 g	Cholesterol:	0 mg	Potassium:	284 mg
Protein:	6 g	Fiber:	5.7 g	Calcium:	35 mg
Total Fat:	3 g	Sodium:	143 mg	Iron:	1.6 mg

CABBAGE SOUP

(dairy-free, egg-free, gluten-free)   *Makes 8 servings*

Here's an old-fashioned sweet-and-sour cabbage soup that gets its flavor from beef bones. Sour salt is available in the seasoning section of your market. Yeast-free dieters should omit the vinegar.

INGREDIENTS
1 pound beef bones
2 quarts water
½ teaspoon salt
2 large onions, sliced
1 (28-ounce) can tomatoes in purée
1 medium head cabbage, shredded
2 tablespoons lemon juice
2 tablespoons vinegar
1 tablespoon brown sugar
¼ teaspoon pepper
¼ teaspoon ground ginger
⅛ teaspoon sour salt (citric acid optional)

Place bones in a large, deep soup pot. Add 2 quarts of water and the salt. Bring to a boil. Skim the surface with a large spoon to remove residue. Turn the heat to low and add onions, tomatoes, cabbage, lemon juice, vinegar, sugar, pepper, ginger, and sour salt. Stir. Cook, covered, over low heat for 2 hours. Taste and add additional lemon juice or sugar as needed to obtain the balanced sweet-and-sour taste desired.

NUTRITION PER SERVING

		Calories:	35		
Carbohydrate:	8 g	Cholesterol:	0 mg	Potassium:	274 mg
Protein:	1 g	Fiber:	.6 g	Calcium:	20 mg
Total Fat:	0 g	Sodium:	256 mg	Iron:	.7 mg

CHICKEN SOUP

(dairy-free, egg-free, gluten-free, sugar-free, yeast-free)   *Makes 8 servings*

There are times when you or a friend are going to be sick and just yearn for some of Mama's chicken soup. If Mama didn't show you how to make it, it's here for the learning! Basically, it's just chicken and water with some vegetables to flavor the broth. You can do it!

INGREDIENTS
1 chicken, about 3 pounds
2 quarts water
1 whole onion
2 whole carrots, scraped
4 celery stalks, including leaves
1 parsnip, scraped
2 parsley sprigs
2 dill sprigs
1/2 teaspoon salt
1/4 teaspoon white pepper
4 ounces fine noodles, cooked (optional)

Rinse chicken, remove liver and place rinsed giblets and neck into a large soup pot. Remove any viscera clinging to the chicken. Place chicken in the pot, add 2 quarts of water and the remaining ingredients. Bring to a boil, then simmer over low heat covered until chicken is tender, about 2 hours. Remove chicken and refrigerate separately, pour soup through a strainer, and chill. (Carrots may be cut up and left in the broth, if desired.) Skim off the fat that rises to the top of chilled soup and discard it. Reheat the portion of soup desired. Serve with cooked noodles and pieces of the cooked chicken (skin removed) and carrot.

NUTRITION PER SERVING

		Calories:	104		
Carbohydrate:	9 g	Cholesterol:	66 mg	Potassium:	310 mg
Protein:	12 g	Fiber:	6 g	Calcium:	29 mg
Total Fat:	2 g	Sodium:	198 mg	Iron:	1.2 mg

FISH CHOWDER

(egg-free, gluten-free, sugar-free, yeast-free)   *Makes 8 servings*

How do you feed 8 hungry people when you have only 1 pound of fish to divide among them? Turn it into a tasty chowder.

INGREDIENTS

4 potatoes, peeled and cubed
2 onions, thinly sliced
3 cups water
1 dill sprig
½ teaspoon salt
¼ teaspoon celery salt
¼ teaspoon ground dried thyme
¼ teaspoon pepper
1 pound fish fillets
3 cups skim milk
1 tablespoon corn oil margarine
Paprika to garnish

Place potatoes, onions, water, fresh dill, salt, celery salt, thyme, and pepper in a large saucepan. Cover and cook over low heat 15 minutes, or until potatoes are tender. Cut fish fillets into bite-size chunks and add to the pot. Add milk and margarine. Simmer, covered, for 15 minutes more, or until fish is tender. Ladle into bowls and serve with a dash of paprika on each.

NUTRITION PER SERVING

		Calories:	209		
Carbohydrate:	16 g	Cholesterol:	36 mg	Potassium:	700 mg
Protein:	22 g	Fiber:	4 g	Calcium:	135 mg
Total Fat:	6 g	Sodium:	335 mg	Iron:	1.2 mg

SPLIT PEA SOUP

(*dairy-free, egg-free, gluten-free, sugar-free*)   *Makes 8 servings*

Legumes are an alternate source of protein. If you've ever yearned for a real old-fashioned bowl of split pea soup and want to make your own, here's the way to satisfy your craving. Float some garlic croutons on the top as a garnish.

INGREDIENTS
2 cups dried split peas
2 quarts water
2 meaty beef neck bones, or a ham bone
1 onion, finely diced
2 carrots, scraped and thinly sliced
2 celery stalks, thinly sliced
Several parsley sprigs, fresh, finely cut
Several dill sprigs, fresh, finely cut
3/4 teaspoon salt
1/4 teaspoon pepper

Place split peas in a large heavy saucepan and add the water. Add the remaining ingredients and stir. Bring to a boil, then turn the heat to low, cover and simmer for 2 1/2 to 3 hours. Stir occasionally. To serve, remove the bones and strain the soup through a food mill, if smooth soup is desired. Otherwise, serve as it is with bits of meat from the bones.

NUTRITION PER SERVING, WITH BITS OF MEAT

			Calories:	181		
Carbohydrate:	35 g	Cholesterol:	8 mg	Potassium:	672 mg
Protein:	11 g	Fiber:	2.7 g	Calcium:	89 mg
Total Fat:	.8 g	Sodium:	258 mg	Iron:	2.7 mg

HEARTY VEGETABLE SOUP

(dairy-free, egg-free, gluten-free, sugar-free)   *Makes 8 servings*

Soup is a comfort food. Don't be restricted by the list of vegetables in this recipe—add whatever extra vegetables you may have in the refrigerator that seem to be limp. A sprinkling of diced left-over chicken or beef heated in a portion of the soup would make it a meal-in-one. Gluten-free dieters should use rice instead of barley.

INGREDIENTS
1/2 cup white navy beans
3 beef marrow bones, optional
2 quarts water
1 large yellow turnip, peeled and diced
3 large onions, sliced
4 carrots, scraped and sliced
4 celery stalks with leaves, sliced
3 tomatoes, quartered, or 1 (16-ounce) can tomatoes
1/2 cup barley or rice
2 bay leaves
1/2 teaspoon salt
1/4 teaspoon pepper
1/4 teaspoon dried thyme
1/4 teaspoon dried oregano

Soak the navy beans in water to cover for several hours; drain. Place all the ingredients into a large soup pot. Add 2 quarts of water and bring to a boil, then lower the heat, cover, and simmer over low heat for 2 hours.

NUTRITION PER SERVING
Calories: 103

Carbohydrate:	23 g	Cholesterol:	0 mg	Potassium:	481 mg
Protein:	3 g	Fiber:	1 g	Calcium:	58 mg
Total Fat:	.2 g	Sodium:	194 mg	Iron:	1.4 mg

14

EASY MAIN ENTRÉES

Ⅰf YOU'VE BEEN LIVING ON FAST FOOD, FRO-
zen dinners, and packaged dehydrated products, chances are you've been
eating a high-fat, high-sodium, refined-nutrients existence. This chapter
will show you how to change your food habits and how to cook fast, simple,
and healthy foods.

It helps to have the basics in your kitchen—onions, garlic, several cans
of tomatoes or tomato purée, and a good assortment of dried herbs. Bake,
broil, or cook in a nonstick skillet—frying in fat can make your food as
soggy as your mood.

All of these recipes were developed for people with a busy lifestyle.
They will give you the opportunity to enjoy good meals without spending
too much time preparing them.

Be sure to rotate your choice of poultry, fish, or meat daily, as well as
your choice of accompanying vegetables and whole grains. When you eat
the same thing every day, you are supplying a very narrow range of nutrients, especially the trace minerals. Those people prone to food sensitivities
should be especially careful in rotating food selections.

Sometimes you can cook and coast, freezing extra portions for another
night when you are crunched for time. It's the way to have good food with
no extra fat or additives—ready to be microwaved or heated in the oven.

BOILED CODFISH

(dairy-free, egg-free, gluten-free, sugar-free)   *Makes 4 servings*

Purchase whatever firm white-fleshed fish is least expensive. Cod is usually in that category. Be sure to include the vinegar if you are not on a yeast-free diet—it helps to firm up the fish.

INGREDIENTS
2 codfish steaks, about 1¼ pounds
1 small onion, diced
1 small carrot, pared and diced
1 parsley sprig
¼ cup tarragon vinegar
1 bay leaf
2 whole cloves

Place fish in a large skillet with a tight cover. Add onion, carrot, and parsley. Cover fish with water and add vinegar, bay leaf, and cloves. Bring quickly to a boil, then cover and reduce the heat to keep the liquid just below the boiling point. Simmer for 10 minutes, or until fish flakes easily.

NUTRITION PER SERVING

		Calories:	300		
Carbohydrate:	5 g	Cholesterol:	108 mg	Potassium:	942 mg
Protein:	43 g	Fiber:	.3 g	Calcium:	47 mg
Total Fat:	11 g	Sodium:	344 mg	Iron:	2.4 mg

BAKED COD TARRAGON

(dairy-free, egg-free, gluten-free, sugar-free, yeast-free)   *Makes 4 servings*

It's so simple to prepare fish well. Here's a cod dish with a dash of tarragon and a hint of lemon. Be careful not to overcook it!

INGREDIENTS
2 teaspoons salad oil
4 cod fillets, about 1¼ pounds
½ teaspoon paprika
1 small onion, diced
1 garlic clove, minced
3 tomatoes, finely chopped
¼ teaspoon dried tarragon

⅛ teaspoon pepper
¼ cup lemon juice

Brush salad oil over all sides of cod fillets; arrange in one layer in a nonstick baking dish and sprinkle with paprika. Combine onion, garlic, tomatoes, tarragon, pepper, and lemon juice in a small saucepan; cook and stir for several minutes. Pour sauce over fish. Bake in a 350° F oven for 30 minutes, or until fish flakes easily.

NUTRITION PER SERVING

		Calories:	240		
Carbohydrate:	7 g	Cholesterol:	108 mg	Potassium:	729 mg
Protein:	33 g	Fiber:	.6 g	Calcium:	51 mg
Total Fat:	8 g	Sodium:	129 mg	Iron:	1.6 mg

BAKED FISH ESPAÑOL

(dairy-free, egg-free, sugar-free)   *Makes 2 servings*

*Fish takes kindly to delicate vegetables and wine during baking. Here's a
Spanish version that will become a favorite once tried. Gluten-free and yeast-free
dieters can omit the bread crumbs.*

INGREDIENTS
2 codfish fillets, about ¾ pound
⅛ teaspoon salt
Dash of pepper
⅛ teaspoon nutmeg
2 slices of onion
2 thick slices tomato
1 tablespoon chopped pimiento
2 tablespoons bread crumbs

Place fish in the bottom of a nonstick baking dish. Sprinkle with salt, pepper, and nutmeg. Separate onion rings and pile on top of fish. Top with tomato and chopped pimiento. Sprinkle with bread crumbs. Bake uncovered in a 350° F oven for 25 minutes, or until fish flakes easily.

NUTRITION PER SERVING

		Calories:	339		
Carbohydrate:	6 g	Cholesterol:	93 mg	Potassium:	887 mg
Protein:	47 g	Fiber:	.2 g	Calcium:	49 mg
Total Fat:	13 g	Sodium:	539 mg	Iron:	2.5 mg

BROILED FLOUNDER PARMESAN

(egg-free, gluten-free, sugar-free, yeast-free)   *Makes 3 servings*

Don't underestimate the flavor power of some chopped fresh tomato. Here it is used as a topping for a simple flounder dish that is good enough for company fare.

INGREDIENTS
1 pound flounder fillets
1/8 teaspoon salt
Dash of pepper
1 tomato, peeled and chopped
1 tablespoon grated onion
1/4 teaspoon oregano
1 tablespoon grated Parmesan cheese

Arrange flounder fillets on a broiling pan. Season with salt and pepper. Spoon chopped tomato over the fillets; sprinkle onion, oregano, and then the grated cheese over the fish. Broil for 10 to 15 minutes, 3 inches below broiler unit, or until fish flakes easily. Do not turn the fish.

NUTRITION PER SERVING
Calories: 324

Carbohydrate:	2 g	Cholesterol:	95 mg	Potassium:	995 mg
Protein:	46 g	Fiber:	.3 g	Calcium:	69 mg
Total Fat:	13 g	Sodium:	464 mg	Iron:	2.4 mg

FLOUNDER WITH SPINACH-SARDINE STUFFING

(dairy-free, egg-free, gluten-free, sugar-free, yeast-free)   *Makes 4 servings*

Sardines are a good source of calcium. Here's a novel way to serve them. Yeast-free dieters should omit the wine.

INGREDIENTS
4 flounder fillets, about 1 pound
1 tablespoon lime juice
1 (10-ounce) package frozen chopped spinach, thawed
1 (4-ounce) can sardines with bones, drained and mashed
1 tablespoon grated onion
1/4 teaspoon nutmeg

¼ cup lemon juice
¼ cup white wine or water

Sprinkle the fillets with lime juice. In a small bowl, combine spinach, sardines, onion, and nutmeg. Spread spinach mixture in a thin layer over each of the fish fillets. Roll up. Place fish rolls in a large skillet. Pour lemon juice and wine over all. Cook over low heat for 7 minutes, or until fish flakes easily.

NUTRITION PER SERVING

		Calories:	287		
Carbohydrate:	3 g	Cholesterol:	72 mg	Potassium:	962 mg
Protein:	40 g	Fiber:	.3 g	Calcium:	162 mg
Total Fat:	11 g	Sodium:	467 mg	Iron:	3.3 mg

FISH CREOLE

(dairy-free, egg-free, gluten-free, sugar-free, yeast-free)   *Makes 5 servings*

You may prefer to cook your fish with a tomato-based zesty sauce. Here's a way to get dinner on the table in less than 15 minutes.

INGREDIENTS
1 pound flounder or haddock fillets
1 small onion, diced
1 green pepper, diced
1 (8-ounce) can marinara sauce
¼ teaspoon dried thyme
⅛ teaspoon pepper

Place fish in a large skillet. Arrange onion and green pepper around it. Pour marinara sauce over all. Sprinkle with thyme and pepper. Cover and cook over low heat for 10 minutes, or until fish flakes easily.

NUTRITION PER SERVING

		Calories:	332		
Carbohydrate:	6 g	Cholesterol:	72 mg	Potassium:	1,136 mg
Protein:	46 g	Fiber:	.7 g	Calcium:	45 mg
Total Fat:	12 g	Sodium:	467 mg	Iron:	2.7 mg

SOLE FLORENTINE

(dairy-free, egg-free, gluten-free, sugar-free, yeast-free)   *Makes 4 servings*

A bed of seasoned fresh spinach topped with fillet of sole cooks in a matter of minutes. So easy and so satisfying too!

INGREDIENTS
1 pound fresh spinach
1/4 teaspoon nutmeg
1/8 teaspoon pepper
4 sole fillets, about 1 pound
Juice of 1 lemon
Paprika

Wash spinach and rinse until water is clear. Trim well. Place spinach, with plenty of water still clinging to the leaves, in a large nonstick skillet. Cover and cook over low heat for several minutes until spinach wilts. Sprinkle with nutmeg and pepper. Top with slices of sole. Squeeze lemon juice over all. Sprinkle fish with paprika. Cover again and cook over low heat 5 minutes, adding a small amount of extra water if needed. Serve each sole fillet on a bed of spinach.

NUTRITION PER SERVING

		Calories:	250		
Carbohydrate:	3 g	Cholesterol:	72 mg	Potassium:	968 mg
Protein:	36 g	Fiber:	.5 g	Calcium:	110 mg
Total Fat:	9.7 g	Sodium:	314 mg	Iron:	3.6 mg

POACHED FISH ROLLS WITH CHEESE STUFFING

(egg-free, gluten-free, sugar-free, yeast-free)   *Makes 4 servings*

The cheese stuffing creates a delicate balance of flavors with the fish. Keep the heat very low or the milk will scorch.

INGREDIENTS
4 sole fillets, about 1 pound
1/2 cup 1 percent low-fat cottage cheese
1 teaspoon dried dill
1 teaspoon dried chopped chives
1/4 teaspoon paprika
1 cup skim milk

Spread fillets of sole with combined cottage cheese, dill, and chives. Roll up fillets and place in a small nonstick skillet. Sprinkle with paprika. Pour milk around fish rolls. Cover tightly and cook over very low heat for 12 minutes, or until fish flakes easily.

NUTRITION PER SERVING

		Calories:	271		
Carbohydrate:	4 g	Cholesterol:	2 mg	Potassium:	791 mg
Protein:	39 g	Fiber:	0 g	Calcium:	119 mg
Total Fat:	9 g	Sodium:	300 mg	Iron:	1.7 mg

CELERY STUFFED FISH

(dairy-free, egg-free, gluten-free, sugar-free, yeast-free)   *Makes 4 servings*

This stuffing can be used to add fiber and lively flavor to any white-fleshed thin fish fillets such as flounder or sole.

INGREDIENTS
2 tablespoons olive oil
3 cups finely sliced celery
1 small onion, finely diced
1 garlic clove, finely diced
1 (8-ounce) can tomatoes, broken up
2 tablespoons chopped fresh parsley
1/2 teaspoon dried oregano
1/8 teaspoon pepper
4 fish fillets, about 1 pound

Heat oil in a large nonstick skillet. Over low heat, sauté celery, onion, and garlic, stirring constantly, until onion is translucent. Add tomatoes, parsley, oregano, and pepper. Bring to a boil. Remove from heat. Spoon celery mixture on each piece of fish; roll up and place in a nonstick casserole. Spoon remaining celery mixture over and around fish. Cover and bake in a 350° F oven for 25 minutes, or until fish flakes easily.

NUTRITION PER SERVING

		Calories:	320		
Carbohydrate:	8 g	Cholesterol:	72 mg	Potassium:	1,156 mg
Protein:	35 g	Fiber:	1.6 g	Calcium:	76 mg
Total Fat:	16 g	Sodium:	386 mg	Iron:	2.3 mg

BOILED HALIBUT

(*dairy-free, egg-free, gluten-free, sugar-free*)   *Makes 4 servings*

*When boiling or poaching fish, an acid such as vinegar helps firm up the flesh.
Yeast-free dieters may substitute 2 tablespoons lemon juice for the vinegar.*

INGREDIENTS
4 halibut steaks, about 1 pound
1 small onion, diced
1 carrot, scraped and sliced
1 fresh parsley sprig
1 quart water
¼ cup tarragon vinegar
1 tablespoon frozen apple juice concentrate
1 bay leaf
2 whole cloves
2 peppercorns

Arrange fish steaks on the bottom of a large, heavy saucepan, preferably on
a rack. Add onion, carrot, and parsley. Add water, vinegar, apple juice
concentrate, bay leaf, cloves, and peppercorns. Bring quickly to the boiling
point, then lower heat to keep liquid just below boiling. Simmer over low
heat 10 minutes, or until fish flakes easily.

NUTRITION PER SERVING
Calories: 214

Carbohydrate:	5 g	Cholesterol:	72 mg	Potassium:	568 mg
Protein:	33 g	Fiber:	.3 g	Calcium:	48 mg
Total Fat:	6 g	Sodium:	135 mg	Iron:	1.4 mg

BROILED DILLED HALIBUT

(dairy-free, egg-free, gluten-free, sugar-free, yeast-free)   *Makes 3 servings*

Any firm white-fleshed fish will do for this broiled dish. Who says you can't cook fast and healthy?

INGREDIENTS
1 pound halibut fillets
2 tablespoons lemon juice
1/8 teaspoon salt
1/8 teaspoon paprika
1/2 teaspoon dried dill

Arrange fillets on a broiling pan. Sprinkle fish with lemon juice, salt, paprika, and dill. Broil 3 inches from broiler unit for 10 to 12 minutes, or until fish flakes easily when tested with a fork. There is no need to turn the fish over during broiling.

NUTRITION PER SERVING

		Calories:	307		
Carbohydrate:	.6 g	Cholesterol:	72 mg	Potassium:	902 mg
Protein:	45 g	Fiber:	trace	Calcium:	36 mg
Total Fat:	6 g	Sodium:	447 mg	Iron:	2.1 mg

POACHED SALMON

(*dairy-free, egg-free, gluten-free, sugar-free*)   *Makes 2 servings*

The secret to poaching fish properly is to bring the liquid to a boil, then simmer until fish is just opaque. Test with a fork after a few minutes. This is fast food at its best! Yeast-free dieters may substitute 2 tablespoons lemon juice for the vinegar.

INGREDIENTS
2 thin center slices fresh salmon, about ²/₃ pound
1 cup water
¹/₄ cup cider vinegar
1 onion, thinly sliced
1 fresh dill sprig
3 whole cloves
1 bay leaf
1 peppercorn
2 lemon wedges

Place salmon slices in a large skillet. Add water, vinegar, onion, dill, cloves, bay leaf, and peppercorn. Bring to a boil, then reduce heat and simmer, covered, 6 to 10 minutes, or until salmon is cooked through. Remove with a slotted spatula. Serve garnished with lemon wedges, and additional dill sprigs.

NUTRITION PER SERVING
		Calories:	190		
Carbohydrate:	6 g	Cholesterol:	90 mg	Potassium:	497 mg
Protein:	24 g	Fiber:	.2 g	Calcium:	235 mg
Total Fat:	7 g	Sodium:	442 mg	Iron:	1.4 mg

SALMON LOAF

(*dairy-free, sugar-free*)   *Makes 4 servings*

Keep a can of salmon on hand for just that moment when you need to make a pick-of-the-pantry meal. Gluten-free and yeast-free dieters may substitute 1 large grated potato for the bread crumbs.

INGREDIENTS
1 (15¹/₂-ounce) can salmon
¹/₂ cup soft fresh whole-wheat bread crumbs

¼ cup chopped green onions, including tops
2 tablespoons chopped parsley
1 egg white, beaten
⅛ teaspoon pepper
⅛ teaspoon dried tarragon

Drain salmon and flake into a medium bowl. Add bread crumbs, scallions, parsley, and egg white. Add pepper and tarragon. Mix well. Spoon into a nonstick 8 × 4-inch loaf pan. Bake at 350° F for 30 minutes.

NUTRITION PER SERVING
Calories: 210

Carbohydrate:	10 g	Cholesterol:	37 mg	Potassium:	454 mg
Protein:	24 g	Fiber:	.2 g	Calcium:	237 mg
Total Fat:	7 g	Sodium:	528 mg	Iron:	1.5 mg

BAKED WHOLE RED SNAPPER

(dairy-free, egg-free, gluten-free, sugar-free, yeast-free)   *Makes 4 servings*

Occasionally you may be inspired to purchase a whole red snapper and serve it for dinner. This is a delicately flavored fish, and this recipe caters to that quality.

INGREDIENTS
2 tomatoes, thinly sliced
1 onion, thinly sliced
1 tablespoon corn oil margarine
1 lemon cut in thin slices
1 fresh dill sprig
1 whole red snapper, about 2½ pounds, cleaned

Arrange tomatoes and onion in a layer in the bottom of a flat baking dish. Place dots of margarine and some of the lemon slices in the cavity of the fish. Tuck in the dill. Bake in a 350° F oven for 30 minutes, or until fish flakes easily. Serve with remaining lemon slices.

NUTRITION PER SERVING
Calories: 346

Carbohydrate:	6 g	Cholesterol:	91 mg	Potassium:	1,065 mg
Protein:	45 g	Fiber:	5 g	Calcium:	51 mg
Total Fat:	14 g	Sodium:	387 mg	Iron:	2.5 mg

TUNA-LENTIL CREOLE

(dairy-free, egg-free, gluten-free, yeast-free)   *Makes 6 servings*

Don't overlook lentils as a good source of protein. You can shorten the cooking time by soaking the lentils overnight. If you can find fresh okra, so much the better! Hypoglycemics and yeast-free dieters should omit the brown sugar.

INGREDIENTS
1 cup dried lentils
1 (28-ounce) can tomatoes
1 cup chopped green pepper
³/₄ cup chopped onion
1 package frozen sliced okra, thawed
1 teaspoon brown sugar
¹/₈ teaspoon hot pepper sauce
2 (7-ounce) cans water-packed tuna, drained

Place lentils in a medium saucepan; cover with water. Bring to a boil. Cook uncovered over medium heat for 1¹/₂ hours, adding more water if necessary. Drain and set aside. Place drained juice from tomatoes in a large saucepan. Add green pepper, onion, and okra. Cook 3 minutes over medium heat, stirring occasionally. Add tomatoes, brown sugar, hot pepper sauce, and drained cooked lentils. Cover and simmer 30 minutes. Add flaked tuna and simmer until heated through. Serve over cooked rice, if desired.

NUTRITION PER SERVING

		Calories:	197		
Carbohydrate:	22 g	Cholesterol:	103 mg	Potassium:	704 mg
Protein:	25 g	Fiber:	1.8 g	Calcium:	58 mg
Total Fat:	.3 g	Sodium:	188 mg	Iron:	3.4 mg

SHRIMP PORTUGAISE

(dairy-free, egg-free, gluten-free, sugar-free, yeast-free)   *Makes 4 servings*

You may be able to purchase cooked and cleaned shrimp from your fish market to save time with this dish. It costs a bit more, but saves on effort. The subtle orange flavor makes this a taste treat.

INGREDIENTS
1 cup uncooked rice
2 cups water
1¼ cup orange juice
½ teaspoon salt
1 tablespoon olive oil
1 onion, thinly sliced
1 green pepper, seeded and diced
2 tablespoons chopped pimiento (optional)
1 (8-ounce) can tomato sauce
½ teaspoon grated orange rind
1½ pounds shrimp, cooked, shelled, and deveined
1 whole orange, peeled and broken into segments

Combine rice, water, ½ cup of the orange juice, and ¼ teaspoon of the salt in a large saucepan. Bring to a boil, cover, and reduce the heat. Cook over low heat for 25 minutes, or until the rice is done. Fluff once during the cooking time. Meanwhile, heat oil in a large nonstick skillet. Add onion and green pepper; sauté over medium heat until vegetables are limp. Add pimiento. Stir in tomato sauce, ¾ cup of the orange juice, the orange rind, and ¼ teaspoon of the salt. Bring to a boil; reduce the heat and simmer about 5 minutes. Add shrimp to the tomato mixture and cook just long enough to heat shrimp through. Serve shrimp and sauce on the cooked rice and garnish with orange segments.

NUTRITION PER SERVING

		Calories:	326		
Carbohydrate:	53 g	Cholesterol:	99 mg	Potassium:	526 mg
Protein:	17 g	Fiber:	.7 g	Calcium:	87 mg
Total Fat:	4 g	Sodium:	411 mg	Iron:	3 mg

SHRIMP CREOLE

(dairy-free, egg-free, gluten-free, sugar-free)   *Makes 4 servings*

This shrimp creole dish may be cooked in advance, refrigerated, and reheated just before serving time. You can easily double or triple the recipe to serve a crowd. It takes about 15 minutes to peel and devein 1 pound of medium-size shrimp, so gauge your time accordingly. Yeast-free dieters should use lemon juice instead of vinegar.

INGREDIENTS

1½ pounds shrimp
2 onions, sliced
4 celery stalks, sliced
2 garlic cloves, minced
2 tablespoons olive oil
1 tablespoon cornstarch
½ teaspoon salt
1 tablespoon chili powder
1 cup water
1 (16-ounce) can whole tomatoes
2 cups peas, fresh or frozen
1 tablespoon vinegar

Remove the shells from the shrimp, devein, and rinse thoroughly. In a 2-quart saucepan over medium heat, sauté the onions, celery, and garlic in olive oil, until limp, about 7 minutes. Combine cornstarch, salt, chili powder, and water in a small bowl. Add chili powder mixture to the saucepan. Simmer over low heat, uncovered, stirring occasionally, for 10 minutes. Add tomatoes, peas, vinegar, and shrimp. Simmer for 10 minutes, or until shrimp are tender and pink. Do not overcook because shrimp will get tough.

NUTRITION PER SERVING

Calories: 228

Carbohydrate:	21 g	Cholesterol:	99 mg	Potassium:	684 mg
Protein:	18 g	Fiber:	2 g	Calcium:	89 mg
Total Fat:	7 g	Sodium:	655 mg	Iron:	3.5 mg

SAUTÉED OYSTERS

(dairy-free, egg-free, gluten-free, sugar-free, yeast-free)   *Makes 2 servings*

If you are an oyster lover, you're adding extra iron to your diet whenever you eat them. If they are in season, buy a pint of freshly shucked oysters to serve two people. They'll be cooked before you set the table!

INGREDIENTS
1 tablespoon corn oil margarine
1 pint freshly shucked oysters with liquid
2 tablespoons finely chopped celery
2 tablespoons finely chopped green pepper
1 tablespoon finely chopped fresh parsley
2 teaspoons lemon juice
1/4 teaspoon salt
1/8 teaspoon pepper

Melt margarine in a large skillet, then add oysters and liquid. Add celery, green pepper, parsley, lemon juice, salt, and pepper. Cook and stir until the edges of the oysters begin to curl, about 2 to 3 minutes.

NUTRITION PER SERVING

		Calories:	213		
Carbohydrate:	9 g	Cholesterol:	120 mg	Potassium:	356 mg
Protein:	20 g	Fiber:	.2 g	Calcium:	237 mg
Total Fat:	9 g	Sodium:	521 mg	Iron:	13 mg

POACHED DILLED SCALLOPS

(dairy-free, egg-free, gluten-free, sugar-free)   *Makes 4 servings*

When you need fast food, poach scallops in a skillet. They cook in minutes while you prepare the vegetables. Yeast-free dieters should omit the wine and substitute water instead.

INGREDIENTS
1 pound fresh scallops
$\frac{1}{2}$ cup white wine
2 tablespoons lemon juice
1 fresh dill sprig
2 peppercorns

Wash scallops and pat dry. Place scallops in a skillet. Add wine, lemon juice, dill, and peppercorns. Cover and cook over low heat for 5 to 8 minutes, or until cooked through. Do not overcook or the scallops will get tough.

NUTRITION PER SERVING
Calories: 129

Carbohydrate:	.5 g	Cholesterol:	40 mg	Potassium:	550 mg
Protein:	26 g	Fiber:	trace	Calcium:	131 mg
Total Fat:	6 g	Sodium:	300 mg	Iron:	3.4 mg

APRICOT BROILED CHICKEN

(dairy-free, egg-free, gluten-free, sugar-free, yeast-free)   *Makes 4 servings*

Except for the skin, chicken is a good source of low-fat protein. Here it is broiled sweet and easy.

INGREDIENTS
1 broiler chicken, quartered, about 3 pounds
6 unsweetened apricot halves, may be canned
$\frac{1}{2}$ teaspoon dry mustard
$\frac{1}{4}$ teaspoon dried oregano
$\frac{1}{8}$ teaspoon pepper

Arrange chicken pieces on a broiler pan. Purée apricot halves, dry mustard, oregano, and pepper in an electric blender; spread thinly over chicken.

Broil 3 inches from heat 10 minutes on each side, or until done. Remove skin before eating.

NUTRITION PER SERVING

		Calories:	231		
Carbohydrate:	8 g	Cholesterol:	60 mg	Potassium:	497 mg
Protein:	37 g	Fiber:	.3 g	Calcium:	21 mg
Total Fat:	5 g	Sodium:	55 mg	Iron:	1.7 mg

CHICKEN TERIYAKI

(dairy-free, egg-free, gluten-free)   *Makes 4 servings*

When you are in a hurry, use this tasty way of broiling chicken. Low-sodium soy sauce is available in most health-food stores. Yeast-dieters should omit this one because of soy sauce and sugar. The recipe is okay for hypoglycemics, but they should omit the sugar.

INGREDIENTS
4 boneless chicken breast halves, skinned
¼ cup low-sodium soy sauce
½ teaspoon ground ginger
1 garlic clove, minced
1 teaspoon brown sugar

Place chicken on a broiling rack. Combine soy sauce, ginger, garlic, and brown sugar in a small bowl; brush half the mixture on top of chicken. Broil 3 inches from heat for 10 minutes. Turn and brush remaining sauce on top of chicken. Broil 5 to 10 minutes more, until chicken is cooked through.

NUTRITION PER SERVING

		Calories:	209		
Carbohydrate:	1 g	Cholesterol:	60 mg	Potassium:	269 mg
Protein:	36 g	Fiber:	trace	Calcium:	14 mg
Total Fat:	5 g	Sodium:	51 mg	Iron:	1.5 mg

BROILED CHICKEN PIQUANT

(dairy-free, egg-free, gluten-free, sugar-free, yeast-free)   *Makes 4 servings*

Vegetable oil, such as corn oil, does not have the cholesterol content of butter. Here it is used to keep the chicken moist throughout broiling. The herbs give all a zing of extra flavor!

INGREDIENTS
1 broiler chicken, quartered, about 3 pounds
¼ teaspoon salt
⅛ teaspoon pepper
1 tablespoon salad oil
¼ cup lemon juice
1 tablespoon grated onion
½ teaspoon dried rosemary
½ teaspoon dried tarragon

Sprinkle chicken with salt and pepper and place on a broiling pan. Combine oil, lemon juice, onion, rosemary, and tarragon in a small bowl. Brush chicken with half the lemon juice mixture. Broil 3 to 4 inches from heat, skin side up, for 7 minutes. Turn and brush remainder of lemon juice mixture over chicken. Broil an additional 7 to 10 minutes, or until chicken is done. To test for doneness, the leg should twist easily out of thigh joint and the meat should be fork tender. Remove skin before eating.

NUTRITION PER SERVING
Calories: 154

Carbohydrate:	1.5 g	Cholesterol:	131 mg	Potassium:	267 mg
Protein:	21 g	Fiber:	.02 g	Calcium:	11 mg
Total Fat:	6.7 g	Sodium:	192 mg	Iron:	1.5 mg

CHILI CHICKEN

(dairy-free, egg-free, gluten-free, yeast-free)   *Makes 4 servings*

When you want a barbecued flavor, use this method of marinating chicken in its own sauce. This may be made without the molasses, if desired.

INGREDIENTS
1 broiler chicken, skinned, quartered, about 3 pounds
1 (8-ounce) can tomato sauce
1 teaspoon prepared mustard
1 teaspoon molasses
1 teaspoon chili powder
1 garlic clove, crushed
1 small onion, grated

Place chicken parts in a zipper locking plastic bag. Combine remaining ingredients in a small bowl; pour over chicken into the bag. Refrigerate for several hours. Arrange the chicken on a broiling pan or an outdoor barbecue. Baste chicken with marinade before broiling. When browned on one side (about 10 minutes), turn and baste other side. Broil until done, basting again as needed.

NUTRITION PER SERVING
		Calories:	142		
Carbohydrate:	5 g	Cholesterol:	131 mg	Potassium:	427 mg
Protein:	22 g	Fiber:	.4 g	Calcium:	22 mg
Total Fat:	3 g	Sodium:	61 mg	Iron:	1.9 mg

CHICKEN WITH LEMON YOGURT SAUCE

(egg-free, gluten-free, sugar-free, yeast-free)   *Makes 4 servings*

Here's a quick trick to cook chicken breasts with an intriguing sauce. Cholesterol watchers will love it!

INGREDIENTS
4 boneless skinless chicken breast halves
1/4 cup lemon juice
1/2 teaspoon paprika
1/2 cup water
1 parsley sprig
1/4 cup lemon low-fat yogurt

Sprinkle chicken with lemon juice. Arrange chicken in a large nonstick skillet. Sprinkle with paprika. Add water and parsley. Cover and simmer over low heat for 15 minutes, or until cooked through. Remove chicken to a warm platter. Stir yogurt into the cooking broth, then cook and stir; use low heat to prevent curdling. Pour over chicken and serve.

NUTRITION PER SERVING
Calories: 215

Carbohydrate:	3 g	Cholesterol:	60 mg	Potassium:	411 mg
Protein:	37 g	Fiber:	.03 g	Calcium:	43 mg
Total Fat:	5.2 g	Sodium:	55 mg	Iron:	1.6 mg

CHICKEN WITH PINEAPPLE-PEPPER SAUCE

(dairy-free, egg-free, gluten-free, sugar-free, yeast-free)   *Makes 4 servings*

You can cook chicken breasts in a skillet, poaching them in unsweetened juice. This way is fast and fancy.

INGREDIENTS
4 chicken breast halves, boned and skinned
1 (16-ounce) can pineapple tidbits in natural juice
1/4 cup finely chopped onion
1/4 cup finely chopped green pepper
1/4 cup finely chopped celery
1/2 teaspoon grated lemon rind
1/4 teaspoon ground ginger

¹/₄ teaspoon nutmeg
¹/₈ teaspoon pepper

Arrange chicken breasts in a large nonstick skillet. Pour pineapple, including juice, around chicken. Add onion, green pepper, celery, grated lemon rind, ginger, nutmeg, and pepper. Cover and simmer over low heat 15 to 20 minutes, or until chicken is tender. Add a small amount of water, if needed. Serve over hot cooked rice, if desired.

NUTRITION PER SERVING

		Calories:	255		
Carbohydrate:	14 g	Cholesterol:	60 mg	Potassium:	521 mg
Protein:	37 g	Fiber:	.9 g	Calcium:	33 mg
Total Fat:	5 g	Sodium:	67 mg	Iron:	2 mg

COQ AU VIN

(dairy-free, egg-free, gluten-free)   *Makes 4 servings*

Cook some broad noodles about 15 minutes before serving time and add to the pot, if desired. As it is, it's gluten-free. Wine evaporates during cooking but substitute bouillon for it if you are on a yeast-free diet. Serve with a sprig of dill, if possible. Mighty good eating!

INGREDIENTS
1 broiler chicken, about 3 pounds, cut up
¹/₂ teaspoon salt
¹/₄ teaspoon pepper
1 (16-ounce) can tomatoes
1 onion, thinly sliced
¹/₂ cup burgundy wine, or other dry red wine
1 tablespoon lemon juice
¹/₄ teaspoon dried thyme

Place chicken parts in a heavy casserole. Season with salt and pepper. Add tomatoes, onion, wine, lemon juice, and thyme. Cover tightly. Bake in a 350° oven for 1 hour, or until tender. Remove skin before eating.

NUTRITION PER SERVING

		Calories:	173		
Carbohydrate:	7 g	Cholesterol:	131 mg	Potassium:	554 mg
Protein:	22 g	Fiber:	.6 g	Calcium:	23 mg
Total Fat:	3 g	Sodium:	483 mg	Iron:	2.3 mg

CHICKEN PROVENÇALE

(dairy-free, egg-free, gluten-free, sugar-free, yeast-free)   *Makes 4 servings*

The ingredients for the sauce may be easily doubled or tripled to serve more people or to store in the freezer for those dinners when you'd like to coast on past efforts. Add other chicken parts, if you prefer. Figure on serving 2 thighs per person with this recipe.

INGREDIENTS
8 chicken thighs
1 tablespoon olive oil
1 small onion, thinly sliced
1 garlic clove, minced
1 (16-ounce) can tomatoes, packed in sauce
1/4 teaspoon salt
1/4 teaspoon dried oregano
1/4 teaspoon dried rosemary
1/8 teaspoon dried thyme

Rinse chicken parts and wipe dry with paper towels. Heat oil in a large skillet; sauté over low heat onion and garlic until limp. Add chicken and brown lightly on all sides. Pour off excess oil. Add tomatoes over all. Add salt, oregano, rosemary, and thyme. Cover and simmer for 45 minutes, or until tender. Remove skin from chicken before eating.

NUTRITION PER SERVING

		Calories:	242		
Carbohydrate:	8 g	Cholesterol:	60 mg	Potassium:	282 mg
Protein:	27 g	Fiber:	.8 g	Calcium:	23 mg
Total Fat:	10 g	Sodium:	291 mg	Iron:	2.7 mg

STEWED CHICKEN

(dairy-free, egg-free, gluten-free, sugar-free)   *Makes 4 servings*

Do you yearn for simple cooked chicken-in-the-pot, with noodles and enough liquid to serve it in a soup bowl? Here's the answer and oh-so-easy to do! Yeast-free dieters should omit the wine and the mushrooms.

INGREDIENTS
1 broiler chicken, about 3 pounds
1 (16-ounce) can whole tomatoes
1 chicken bouillon cube
1 cup boiling water
1 onion, thinly sliced
1 green pepper, diced
1/2 pound fresh mushrooms, sliced
1/2 teaspoons salt
1/4 teaspoon pepper
1/4 teaspoon paprika
1/2 cup dry white wine
1 fresh dill sprig, or 1 teaspoon dried

Place chicken in a Dutch oven or heavy pot with lid. Add giblets and neck. Add tomatoes with their juice. Add bouillon cube mixed with boiling water. Add onion, green pepper, and mushrooms. Sprinkle salt, pepper, and paprika over all. Pour wine over all. Add dill. Cover the pot and simmer over low heat for 1 hour, or until chicken can be pierced easily with a fork. Overcooked chicken will fall away from the bones. Spoon broth over chicken occasionally during cooking to keep it moist. Remove skin from chicken before eating.

NUTRITION PER SERVING
Calories: 182

Carbohydrate:	9 g	Cholesterol:	132 mg	Potassium:	662 mg
Protein:	23 g	Fiber:	1 g	Calcium:	26 mg
Total Fat:	3 g	Sodium:	729 mg	Iron:	2.5 mg

CHICKEN CACCIATORE

(dairy-free, egg-free, gluten-free, sugar-free)   *Makes 4 servings*

If this is one of the dishes you frequently order in restaurants and never dreamed you could make at home, give it a try. Yours may be infinitely better! Yeast-free dieters should omit the mushrooms.

INGREDIENTS
$\frac{1}{2}$ teaspoon salt
$\frac{1}{8}$ teaspoon pepper
1 broiler chicken, cut in parts, about 3 pounds
2 tablespoons olive oil
1 onion, thinly sliced
1 green pepper, finely chopped
1 garlic clove, minced
1 chicken bouillon cube
1 cup boiling water
1 (16-ounce) can tomatoes
$\frac{1}{2}$ pound fresh mushrooms, sliced
$\frac{1}{2}$ teaspoon dried oregano

Sprinkle salt and pepper over chicken parts. Heat oil in a large nonstick skillet; brown pieces of chicken over medium heat, turning frequently to brown all sides. Add onion, green pepper, and garlic; stir for several minutes over low heat. Combine bouillon cube and boiling water; add to chicken. Add tomatoes, mushrooms, and oregano. Stir and cover. Simmer over low heat for 1 hour, or until chicken is easily pierced with a fork.

NUTRITION PER SERVING

Calories: 221

Carbohydrate:	9 g	Cholesterol:	132 mg	Potassium:	666 mg
Protein:	23 g	Fiber:	1 g	Calcium:	26 mg
Total Fat:	10 g	Sodium:	729 mg	Iron:	2.5 mg

CHICKEN FRICASSEE

(*dairy-free, egg-free, gluten-free, sugar-free, yeast-free*)   *Makes 8 servings*

This recipe is for those days when you feel like puttering around the kitchen to get old-fashioned flavors the long cooking way. Well worth the effort!

INGREDIENTS

Wings, thighs, legs, and backs of 2 chickens
2 medium onions, diced
2 tablespoons corn oil
1 cup boiling chicken broth (may be made from bouillon cubes)
1 pound lean ground beef
1 egg, beaten
1 tablespoon chopped parsley
1 small onion, grated
1/2 teaspoon salt
1/4 teaspoon pepper
1 tablespoon cornstarch
1/4 cup cold water

Sauté chicken parts and diced onions in the oil in a deep saucepan over medium heat, stirring constantly until chicken parts are brown on all sides. Add broth, cover, and simmer. Combine ground beef, egg, water, parsley, grated onion, salt, and pepper in a medium bowl. Form tiny meatballs and add to chicken. Cook for 30 minutes over very low heat. To thicken the broth, combine 1 tablespoon of cornstarch with 1/4 cup cold water, mix well to form a smooth paste, add 2 tablespoons of hot broth from the chicken to this mixture and then pour all back into the pot while stirring. Stir until a boiling point is reached and broth thickens. Add additional salt and pepper to taste. Remove skin before eating.

NUTRITION PER SERVING

		Calories:	235		
Carbohydrate:	3 g	Cholesterol:	171 mg	Potassium:	365 mg
Protein:	29 g	Fiber:	.2 g	Calcium:	23 mg
Total Fat:	12 g	Sodium:	333 mg	Iron:	2.9 mg

CHICKEN AND PEPPERS

(dairy-free, egg-free, gluten-free, sugar-free, yeast-free)   *Makes 4 servings*

The extra sauce in this dish will go well on pasta or rice. Time your cooking so all is done at the same time.

INGREDIENTS

1 broiler chicken, cut into parts, about 3 pounds
1 tablespoon olive oil
2 large green peppers, sliced into strips
1 onion, thinly sliced
1 garlic clove, minced
3 tomatoes, coarsely chopped
1 cup tomato juice
1/2 teaspoon dried oregano
1/4 teaspoon dried rosemary
1/8 teaspoon pepper

In a large nonstick skillet over medium heat, brown chicken parts in oil. Pour off any remaining oil. Add the remaining ingredients. Cover and cook over low heat for 45 minutes, or until chicken parts are tender. Remove skin before eating.

NUTRITION PER SERVING

Calories: 196

Carbohydrate:	11 g	Cholesterol:	131 mg	Potassium:	719 mg
Protein:	23 g	Fiber:	1 g	Calcium:	33 mg
Total Fat:	6 g	Sodium:	68 mg	Iron:	2.8 mg

CHICKEN AND LIMA STEW

(dairy-free, egg-free, gluten-free, sugar-free)   *Makes 4 servings*

Soak the beans overnight if you can. They'll cook faster and be easier to digest. Yeast-free dieters should omit the wine.

INGREDIENTS
1 cup small dried lima beans
8 small chicken thighs, skinned
2 cups chopped tomatoes
4 carrots, scraped, cut into chunks
4 small parsnips, scraped, cut into chunks
1 large onion, thinly sliced
1 cup dry white wine, or water
1 teaspoon dried rosemary
$1/2$ teaspoon dried thyme
$1/4$ teaspoon pepper

Cover lima beans with water and soak several hours or overnight. Place chicken thighs in a Dutch oven or heavy ovenproof pot. Add drained lima beans, tomatoes, carrots, parsnips, and onion. Pour wine over all. Add rosemary, thyme, and pepper. Mix well. Cover tightly and bake in a 350° F oven for $1^{1}/4$ hours, or until tender.

NUTRITION PER SERVING
Calories: 423

Carbohydrate:	45 g	Cholesterol:	60 mg	Potassium:	1,198 mg
Protein:	36 g	Fiber:	4 g	Calcium:	94 mg
Total Fat:	11 g	Sodium:	12 mg	Iron:	6 mg

CHICKEN-TURNIP STEW

(*dairy-free, egg-free, gluten-free, sugar-free, yeast-free*)   *Makes 4 servings*

If you like turnips, you'll love this stew. The hint of rosemary makes it special.

INGREDIENTS
1 garlic clove, finely minced
1 tablespoon olive oil
1 broiler chicken, about 3 pounds, cut in parts
1 large yellow turnip, peeled and cut in chunks
2 white turnips, peeled and cut in chunks
1 onion, thinly sliced
4 carrots, scraped and cut in chunks
4 large potatoes, peeled and cut in chunks
4 celery stalks, cut in chunks
1 1/2 cups chicken broth
2 tablespoons fresh chopped parsley
1/4 teaspoon dried rosemary
1/4 teaspoon dried thyme
1/2 teaspoon salt
1/8 teaspoon pepper

In a large heavy pot over medium heat, sauté garlic in olive oil, stirring constantly. Add chicken parts; cook and stir for a few minutes. Add turnips, onion, carrots, potatoes, and celery. Pour broth over all. Add parsley, rosemary, thyme, salt, and pepper. Mix well. Cover and cook over low heat 1 1/2 hours, or until tender, adding more broth or water if necessary. Remove skin before eating.

NUTRITION PER SERVING
Calories: 260

Carbohydrate:	32 g	Cholesterol:	60 mg	Potassium:	1,120 mg
Protein:	34 g	Fiber:	2 g	Calcium:	80 mg
Total Fat:	3.5 g	Sodium:	307 mg	Iron:	3.1 mg

STEWED BONELESS CHICKEN

(dairy-free, egg-free, gluten-free, sugar-free, yeast-free)   *Makes 4 servings*

Sometimes simple cooking is best of all. Here's the way to cook chicken so it is moist and tender. Leftovers make great chicken salad.

INGREDIENTS
1 broiler chicken, about 3 pounds
3 cups water,
1 cup sliced celery stalks and leaves
1/4 cup chopped fresh parsley
1 medium onion, sliced
1 bay leaf
1/4 teaspoon dried thyme
1/2 teaspoon salt
1/8 teaspoon pepper
3 tablespoons cornstarch

Place chicken in a large kettle. Add water, celery, parsley, onion, bay leaf, thyme, salt, and pepper. Cover and bring to a boil. Then reduce heat and simmer over low heat 1 hour, or until chicken is tender. Remove chicken from the pot and take the meat off the bones. Discard bones and skin. Strain broth and measure; add boiling water, if necessary, to make 3 cups. Return broth to the kettle. Mix together cornstarch and enough cold water to make a thin paste; spoon some of the broth into this and then return all of this mixture to the kettle. Bring to a boil, stirring constantly, until broth is thickened. Add chicken pieces and heat through. Serve over rice or noodles, as desired.

NUTRITION PER SERVING

		Calories:	155		
Carbohydrate:	8 g	Cholesterol:	131 mg	Potassium:	402 mg
Protein:	22 g	Fiber:	.4 g	Calcium:	32 mg
Total Fat:	3 g	Sodium:	10 mg	Iron:	1.9 mg

BAKED ORANGE CHICKEN

(dairy-free, egg-free, gluten-free, sugar-free, yeast-free)   *Makes 4 servings*

How can something so delicious be so easy? Tuck some sweet potatoes in the oven and bake at the same time.

INGREDIENTS
1 broiler chicken, about 3 pounds
1 orange
1 small onion
1 fresh parsley sprig
1/2 teaspoon salt
1/4 teaspoon paprika

Remove any visible fat from the chicken cavity. Place chicken in a small roasting pan. Cut orange in quarters; squeeze the juice over chicken and then place orange quarters in the chicken cavity. Place onion and parsley in the cavity. Sprinkle chicken with salt and paprika. Bake in a 350° F oven for 1 hour. Remove cavity contents before serving. Do not eat the skin.

NUTRITION PER SERVING
Calories: 142

Carbohydrate:	5 g	Cholesterol:	131 mg	Potassium:	336 mg
Protein:	21 g	Fiber:	.3 g	Calcium:	27 mg
Total Fat:	3 g	Sodium:	60 mg	Iron:	1.7 mg

CURRIED BURGUNDY CHICKEN

(dairy-free, egg-free, gluten-free, sugar-free)   *Makes 4 servings*

Curry really gives a kick of flavor to this easy dish. Serve it on a bed of rice, if you wish. The wine evaporates during cooking but yeast-free dieters should omit wine from this recipe and substitute water.

INGREDIENTS
1 broiler chicken, about 3 pounds, quartered
1 garlic clove, minced
1 small onion, finely diced
1 cup chicken broth
1/2 cup burgundy wine
1 teaspoon curry powder

¹/₂ teaspoon salt
¹/₈ teaspoon pepper

Arrange chicken parts in a flat baking dish. Rub chicken with garlic and
onion. Combine broth, wine, curry powder, salt, and pepper; pour over
chicken. Cover tightly and bake 1 hour in a 350° F oven. Remove the skin
before eating.

NUTRITION PER SERVING

		Calories:	125		
Carbohydrate:	1 g	Cholesterol:	131 mg	Potassium:	262 mg
Protein:	21 g	Fiber:	.07 g	Calcium:	11 mg
Total Fat:	3.5 g	Sodium:	562 mg	Iron:	1.5 mg

BAKED CHICKEN OREGANO

(egg-free, gluten-free, sugar-free, yeast-free)   *Makes 4 servings*

*If you are yearning for fried chicken but are careful about fat in your diet, here's
the way to make a crunchy coating. Buttermilk may sound "fat" but it is
actually the fat-free milk product left over from churning butter.*

INGREDIENTS
1 broiler chicken, cut in parts, about 3 pounds
1 cup cornflake crumbs
¹/₂ teaspoon dried oregano
¹/₂ teaspoon garlic powder
¹/₂ teaspoon paprika
¹/₂ cup buttermilk

Wash and dry chicken pieces. Remove all visible excess fat and skin.
Combine cornflake crumbs, oregano, garlic powder, and paprika. Dip
chicken parts first in buttermilk and then in the crumb mixture, coating
well. Place in a single layer in a foil-lined roasting pan. Bake in a 350° F
oven for 1 hour, or until tender.

NUTRITION PER SERVING

		Calories:	156		
Carbohydrate:	7 g	Cholesterol:	133 mg	Potassium:	295 mg
Protein:	22 g	Fiber:	.05 g	Calcium:	44 mg
Total Fat:	3.7 g	Sodium:	161 mg	Iron:	1.5 mg

HAWAIIAN CHICKEN

(dairy-free, egg-free, gluten-free)   *Makes 4 servings*

If you like the tangy taste of sauced chicken, here's an easy way to make boneless chicken breasts into a gourmet delight. Soy sauce is fermented and is therefore not suitable for a yeast-free diet. You may purchase the boneless breasts in your market at a higher price than whole chicken breasts, or skin and bone them yourself with a sharp knife.

INGREDIENTS
4 skinless boneless chicken breast halves
1/4 teaspoon salt
1 (13 1/2-ounce) can pineapple chunks with juice
1 tablespoon cornstarch
1 teaspoon brown sugar
1/4 teaspoon ground ginger
1/4 teaspoon soy sauce

Arrange chicken breasts in a small baking dish and sprinkle with salt. In a small bowl, drain pineapple juice into cornstarch and blend until smooth. Add pineapple chunks, brown sugar, ginger, and soy sauce. Pour over chicken breasts. Bake in a 350° F oven for 25 to 30 minutes, basting occasionally with the sauce in the pan.

NUTRITION PER SERVING
Calories: 252

Carbohydrate:	14 g	Cholesterol:	60 mg	Potassium:	445 mg
Protein:	37 g	Fiber:	.5 g	Calcium:	25 mg
Total Fat:	5 g	Sodium:	322 mg	Iron:	1.8 mg

BAKED LEMON CHICKEN

(dairy-free, egg-free, gluten-free, sugar-free, yeast-free)   *Makes 4 servings*

Cook the chicken with the skin on, removing all visible fat from the cavity. Be sure to avoid eating the skin because fat lurks underneath. This bakes fast and easy!

INGREDIENTS
1 broiler chicken, cut in parts, about 3 pounds
1 tablespoon corn oil margarine, melted

⅓ cup lemon juice
1 teaspoon dried dill
¼ teaspoon salt
⅛ teaspoon pepper
¼ teaspoon paprika

Arrange chicken in a flat baking dish. Combine the margarine, lemon juice, dill, salt, and pepper in a small bowl; pour over chicken parts. Sprinkle paprika over all. Cover with foil or a tight-fitting lid. Bake in a 350° F oven for 45 minutes, or until tender. Uncover the baking dish the last 10 minutes to brown the chicken.

NUTRITION PER SERVING

		Calories:	150		
Carbohydrate:	2 g	Cholesterol:	131 mg	Potassium:	271 mg
Protein:	21 g	Fiber:	trace	Calcium:	11 mg
Total Fat:	6 g	Sodium:	225 mg	Iron:	1.5 mg

OVEN-FRIED CHICKEN THIGHS

(egg-free, sugar-free, yeast-free)   *Makes 4 servings*

When your market has a special price for chicken thighs, buy them. They may be potted, broiled, or oven-fried with ease. Freeze the extra pieces as a hedge against inflation, or for one of those weeks when your budget is on empty.

INGREDIENTS
8 chicken thighs
¼ cup buttermilk
3 tablespoons unbleached flour
1 tablespoon grated Parmesan cheese
½ teaspoon salt
¼ teaspoon paprika

Dip thighs in buttermilk and then in a mixture of flour, cheese, salt, and paprika. Place thighs in a nonstick baking pan. Bake in a 350° F oven for 20 minutes, then turn and bake 15 to 20 minutes longer, or until tender.

NUTRITION PER SERVING

		Calories:	246		
Carbohydrate:	7 g	Cholesterol:	62 mg	Potassium:	30 mg
Protein:	28 g	Fiber:	.02 g	Calcium:	53 mg
Total Fat:	10 g	Sodium:	298 mg	Iron:	2.2 mg

CHICKEN LIVERS AND GRAPEFRUIT

(*dairy-free, egg-free, gluten-free, sugar-free, yeast-free*)   *Makes 4 servings*

This combination is very high in vitamins A and C, plus iron. That spells good nutrition with a dish that is very low in cost.

INGREDIENTS
1 tablespoon olive oil
1 small onion, diced
2 tablespoons fresh chopped parsley
1 pound chicken livers, cut in halves
1/4 teaspoon salt
2 cups grapefruit sections

Heat oil in a large nonstick skillet. Add onion and sauté over low heat until tender. Add parsley, chicken livers, and salt. Cover and simmer over low heat for 10 minutes, turning livers occasionally. Add grapefruit sections and heat for a moment more. Serve at once.

NUTRITION PER SERVING
Calories: 242

Carbohydrate:	10 g	Cholesterol:	340 mg	Potassium:	280 mg
Protein:	30 g	Fiber:	.2 g	Calcium:	29 mg
Total Fat:	8 g	Sodium:	205 mg	Iron:	10 mg

SAUTÉED CHICKEN LIVERS

(*dairy-free, egg-free, gluten-free, sugar-free, yeast-free*)   *Makes 4 servings*

Chicken livers are bursting with good nutrition and are very inexpensive. Sauté them with onions and sliced celery and serve on toast.

INGREDIENTS
1 bouillon cube
1/2 cup water
1 onion, thinly sliced
2 celery stalks, thinly sliced
1 pound chicken livers
1/2 teaspoon garlic powder
1/4 teaspoon salt
1/8 teaspoon pepper

Put bouillon cube in the water and heat in a large skillet over medium heat until dissolved. Add onion and celery and cook until limp. Add chicken livers. Cook for 5 minutes, stirring occasionally, or until livers are done throughout. Remove livers and let broth cook down over high heat until there is a small amount of reduced liquid. Pour over livers and serve.

NUTRITION PER SERVING

		Calories:	196		
Carbohydrate:	5 g	Cholesterol:	340 mg	Potassium:	246 mg
Protein:	31 g	Fiber:	.2 g	Calcium:	23 mg
Total Fat:	5 g	Sodium:	463 mg	Iron:	9.8 mg

TURKEY ROLL LUAU

(dairy-free, egg-free, gluten-free)   *Makes 8 servings*

Turkey is high in the amino acid tryptophan. Here's a fairly reasonable way to serve 8 people. No need to thaw the turkey roll first—just sauce it and roast to tenderness. Yeast-free dieters should omit soy sauce.

INGREDIENTS

1 turkey roll, about 3 pounds
2 tablespoons brown sugar
1 tablespoon cornstarch
1 (8-ounce) can crushed pineapple
1 tablespoon soy sauce
¼ teaspoon ground ginger

Unwrap turkey roll and rinse; pat dry with paper towels. Arrange turkey roll in a roasting pan. In a small saucepan, combine brown sugar and cornstarch; stir in juice drained from crushed pineapple. Stir over high heat until thickened; add soy sauce, ginger, and drained pineapple. Spoon over turkey roll, covering the entire top surface. Bake in a 350° F oven for 2 hours. Slice and serve.

NUTRITION PER SERVING

		Calories:	133		
Carbohydrate:	7 g	Cholesterol:	44 mg	Potassium:	248 mg
Protein:	18 g	Fiber:	.2 g	Calcium:	13 mg
Total Fat:	3 g	Sodium:	342 mg	Iron:	1.2 mg

TURKEY-STUFFED PEPPERS

(dairy-free, egg-free, gluten-free, sugar-free, yeast-free)   *Makes 8 servings*

Look for freshly ground turkey in your meat market. It is a good choice for a lean meal.

INGREDIENTS

1 pound ground turkey breast
1 cup cooked brown rice
1/2 apple, grated
1/4 teaspoon cinnamon
1/8 teaspoon nutmeg
4 large well-shaped green peppers
2 cups tomato juice
2 tablespoons grated onion
1 tablespoon lemon juice
2 tablespoons seedless white raisins

Combine turkey, rice, apple, cinnamon, and nutmeg in a medium bowl. Mix well. Cut green peppers in half lengthwise, remove membranes and seeds, and rinse well. Lightly stuff pepper halves with turkey mixture. Place peppers in a flat baking dish. Combine tomato juice, onion, lemon juice, and raisins; pour around peppers. Cover dish lightly with foil. Bake 1 hour in a 350° F oven.

NUTRITION PER SERVING

Calories: 165

Carbohydrate:	15 g	Cholesterol:	16 mg	Potassium:	501 mg
Protein:	20 g	Fiber:	1 g	Calcium:	14 mg
Total Fat:	2 g	Sodium:	121 mg	Iron:	1.7 mg

TURKEY BALL STEW

(*dairy-free, sugar-free*)   *Makes 6 servings*

These turkey balls are light and fluffy, cooked and served with zesty vegetables. Gluten-free and yeast-free dieters may omit the bread crumbs and use 2 tablespoons of grated potato instead.

INGREDIENTS
1 eggplant, peeled, cut in ½-inch cubes
1 large onion, sliced
1 garlic clove, minced
2 zucchini, thickly sliced
2 green peppers, cut in cubes
1 (28-ounce) can crushed tomatoes
¼ teaspoon dried oregano
¼ teaspoon dried rosemary
½ teaspoon salt
⅛ teaspoon pepper
1 pound ground turkey breast
¼ cup bread crumbs
1 egg white
1 tablespoon grated onion
1 tablespoon chopped fresh parsley

Place eggplant, sliced onion, garlic, zucchini, green peppers, and tomatoes in a Dutch oven or large casserole. Add oregano, rosemary, salt, and pepper. Combine ground turkey, bread crumbs, egg white, grated onion, and parsley in a medium bowl; form into balls and add to pot. Cover with a tight lid or foil. Bake 1 hour in a 350° F oven.

NUTRITION PER SERVING
Calories: 188

Carbohydrate:	12 g	Cholesterol:	21 mg	Potassium:	697 mg
Protein:	28 g	Fiber:	1.3 g	Calcium:	40 mg
Total Fat:	3 g	Sodium:	195 mg	Iron:	2 mg

CHILI-TURKEY TACOS

(dairy-free, egg-free, gluten-free, sugar-free, yeast-free)   *Makes 10 servings*

Use ground veal or lean beef in place of turkey, if desired. Gluten-free dieters should read taco shell label to be sure they contain no wheat.

INGREDIENTS
1 pound ground turkey breast
1/2 cup cooked pinto beans
1 onion, finely diced
1 1/2 teaspoons chili powder
1 (4-ounce) can tomato paste
1/2 cup water
1/2 teaspoon garlic powder
1/2 teaspoon dried basil
10 taco shells

Sauté ground turkey in a nonstick skillet over medium heat, breaking it apart with a fork as it browns. Add pinto beans, onion, chili powder, tomato paste mixed with the water, garlic powder, and basil. Mix well. Cook until thick and tender, about 15 minutes. Spoon mixture into taco shells and serve. Makes 10 servings.

NUTRITION PER TACO

		Calories:	164		
Carbohydrate:	17 g	Cholesterol:	13 mg	Potassium:	327 mg
Protein:	17 g	Fiber:	.7 g	Calcium:	12 mg
Total Fat:	2.8 g	Sodium:	40 mg	Iron:	1.2 mg

VEAL PICCATA

(dairy-free, egg-free, gluten-free, sugar-free, yeast-free)   *Makes 4 servings*

If you like lemon, this is an easy and delicious way to cook veal. Cook just before eating for best results.

INGREDIENTS
1 pound thin veal slices
2 tablespoons unbleached flour
2 tablespoons olive oil
$1/2$ teaspoon salt
$1/8$ teaspoon pepper
1 lemon, thinly sliced
2 tablespoons chopped fresh parsley

Pound veal slices very thin, using a meat mallet or the side of a knife. Dredge veal slices in flour, shaking off excess to leave a fine powdery coating. Heat olive oil in a nonstick skillet over medium heat; sauté veal slices on both sides. Sprinkle with salt and pepper. Add the lemon slices and parsley. Cook for 5 minutes more, shaking the skillet occasionally. Serve at once.

NUTRITION PER SERVING

		Calories:	250		
Carbohydrate:	4 g	Cholesterol:	trace	Potassium:	285 mg
Protein:	22 g	Fiber:	1 g	Calcium:	19 mg
Total Fat:	15 g	Sodium:	321 mg	Iron:	2.8 mg

VEAL MARSALA

(dairy-free, egg-free, sugar-free) *Makes 3 servings*

This is best cooked at the last moment before dinner, but you can have everything ready beforehand. This takes only minutes to cook and serve. The recipe may be multiplied to feed many more. Mushrooms and wine make this recipe unsuitable for the yeast-free dieter.

INGREDIENTS
¾ pound thin veal slices
2 tablespoons unbleached flour
¼ teaspoon salt
⅛ teaspoon pepper
2 tablespoons olive oil
¼ pound fresh mushrooms, sliced
¼ cup Marsala wine

Flatten veal slices with a meat mallet or with the broad side of a knife. Combine flour, salt, and pepper in a small bowl. Dredge veal slices in the flour mixture until all are lightly coated. Heat oil in a nonstick skillet over medium heat. Brown veal on both sides. When the veal is turned over, add mushrooms. Pour Marsala over all, turn temperature to low, and cook for 5 minutes longer. Serve at once.

NUTRITION PER SERVING

		Calories:	299		
Carbohydrate:	6 g	Cholesterol:	6 mg	Potassium:	312 mg
Protein:	22 g	Fiber:	.1 g	Calcium:	13 mg
Total Fat:	17 g	Sodium:	234 mg	Iron:	2.7 mg

VEAL STROGANOFF

(*egg-free, gluten-free, sugar-free*)   *Makes 4 servings*

*Always add the yogurt just before serving and don't permit the mixture to come
to a boil or the sauce may curdle. Yeast-free dieters should omit the wine and
mushrooms.*

INGREDIENTS
1 pound veal round steak
1 tablespoon olive oil
1/2 pound fresh mushrooms, sliced
1 medium onion, thinly sliced
1 tablespoon cornstarch
1/2 teaspoon paprika
1/4 teaspoon dry mustard
1/4 teaspoon salt
1/8 teaspoon pepper
1/4 cup dry white wine
1 cup plain nonfat yogurt
2 cups cooked brown rice

Cut steak into thin strips. Brown steak in oil over medium heat in a large
nonstick skillet, cover and simmer for 5 minutes. Add mushrooms; cover
and simmer over low heat for 10 minutes more. Remove steak and mushrooms to the top of a large simmering double boiler, covered. Add onion
slices to the skillet, adding additional oil if necessary. Sauté onions until
limp. Sprinkle with cornstarch, paprika, mustard, salt, and pepper; stir
well and brown these ingredients together. Then pour white wine in
slowly, stirring constantly. Remove from heat and stir in yogurt just before
serving. Pour mixture over steak and mushrooms and heat through. Do not
allow mixture to boil. Serve over cooked brown rice.

NUTRITION PER SERVING

		Calories:	380		
Carbohydrate:	33 g	Cholesterol:	6 mg	Potassium:	566 mg
Protein:	28 g	Fiber:	2.4 g	Calcium:	140 mg
Total Fat:	12 g	Sodium:	337 mg	Iron:	3.3 mg

VEAL PAPRIKASH

(*dairy-free, egg-free, sugar-free, yeast-free*)   *Makes 8 servings*

Although veal is expensive, cubed shoulder of veal is not. Here's a way to turn several pounds into a succulent dish. Gluten-free dieters may use rice instead of noodles.

INGREDIENTS
2 pounds lean shoulder of veal, cubed
2 tablespoons paprika
3 medium onions, thinly sliced
2 tablespoons chopped fresh parsley
1 green pepper, seeded and finely diced
½ teaspoon salt
2 cups beef bouillon (may be made from cubes)
1½ tablespoons cornstarch
1 (16-ounce) package wide noodles, cooked
½ teaspoon caraway seed (optional)

Put veal into a small Dutch oven or casserole with tight-fitting cover (aluminum foil may be used). Add paprika, and stir to coat the meat well. Add onion slices, parsley, green pepper, and salt. Pour bouillon around the meat. Cover tightly and bake in a 325° F oven for about 2 hours, or until meat is fork tender. Remove casserole from oven. Mix cornstarch with a small amount of water until dissolved into a thin paste; add some of the hot broth to this paste and stir until smooth. Return this mixture to the cooked meat and broth and cook over medium heat on top of the range, stirring constantly, until the broth is slightly thickened. Serve veal on top of noodles that have been sprinkled with caraway seed.

NUTRITION PER SERVING
Calories: 276

Carbohydrate:	22 g	Cholesterol:	6 mg	Potassium:	380 mg
Protein:	25 g	Fiber:	.5 g	Calcium:	30 mg
Total Fat:	9 g	Sodium:	566 mg	Iron:	3.5 mg

HERBED HAMBURGERS

(dairy-free, egg-free, gluten-free, sugar-free)　　　*Makes 4 servings*

Purchase 1 pound of lean ground beef and use ¹/4 pound for each serving. Yeast-dieters should omit the soy sauce. Wrap extra raw hamburgers in plastic wrap and freeze for another day.

INGREDIENTS
1 pound lean ground beef
2 tablespoons grated onion
1 teaspoon soy sauce
¹/2 teaspoon salt
¹/4 teaspoon pepper
¹/4 teaspoon dried marjoram

Combine all ingredients in a medium bowl and form into 4 hamburgers. Broil 3 inches from broiler about 10 minutes, turning once, depending on degree of rareness desired.

NUTRITION PER HAMBURGER

		Calories:	187		
Carbohydrate:	.5 g	Cholesterol:	77 mg	Potassium:	269 mg
Protein:	23 g	Fiber:	.02 g	Calcium:	10 mg
Total Fat:	10 g	Sodium:	584 mg	Iron:	3 mg

MEATBALL RATATOUILLE

(dairy-free, sugar-free)   *Makes 4 servings*

There may be times when you'd like to make this ratatouille (French vegetable stew) without meat and serve it as a side dish, hot or cold. To do so, omit the ingredients and directions for the meatballs and follow the rest of the recipe. Outrageously good either way! Yeast-free dieters should omit the bread in the meatballs.

INGREDIENTS

1 pound lean ground beef
1 small onion, finely grated
$1/2$ teaspoon salt
$1/4$ teaspoon pepper
1 egg
2 slices whole-grain bread
2 garlic cloves, finely minced
1 large onion, diced
2 tablespoons olive oil
4 medium zucchini, sliced into $1/4$-inch-thick rounds
1 medium eggplant, peeled and diced into 1-inch cubes
1 green pepper, diced into 1-inch cubes
1 (16-ounce) can tomatoes
$1/2$ teaspoon salt
$1/4$ teaspoon pepper
$1/4$ teaspoon dried oregano

Combine beef, grated onion, salt, pepper, and egg in a medium bowl. Soak bread in water and shred it into the beef; mix well. Form mixture into 1-inch meatballs. Sauté diced onion and the garlic in hot oil in a large heavy saucepan; add meatballs and brown over medium heat on all sides. Pour off any remaining fat. Add zucchini, eggplant, green pepper, tomatoes, salt, pepper, oregano, and sherry. Mix well. Cook covered over low heat for 45 minutes.

NUTRITION PER SERVING

		Calories:	368		
Carbohydrate:	22 g	Cholesterol:	145 mg	Potassium:	988 mg
Protein:	12 g	Fiber:	2.6 g	Calcium:	102 mg
Total Fat:	18 g	Sodium:	819 mg	Iron:	5.4 mg

BAKED SPINACH MEATBALLS

(gluten-free, sugar-free, yeast-free)   *Makes 6 servings*

This meatball dish is a meal-in-one when served over hot cooked rice or pasta. The spinach is right in the meatballs! Dairy-free dieters should omit the Parmesan cheese.

INGREDIENTS
1½ pounds lean ground beef
½ cup finely chopped onions
1 egg
¼ cup grated Parmesan cheese
1 (10-ounce) package frozen chopped spinach, thawed
½ teaspoon salt
¼ teaspoon pepper
¼ teaspoon garlic powder
1 cup beef broth (may be made with bouillon cube)
1 (8-ounce) can tomato sauce
1 tablespoon cornstarch

Combine beef, onion, egg, and Parmesan cheese in a medium bowl. Drain spinach and mix thoroughly with beef mixture. Add salt, pepper, and garlic powder; mix well. Form into 1-inch balls. Place into a heavy casserole with a tight lid. Combine broth, tomato sauce, and cornstarch in a small bowl; mix well and pour over meatballs. Cover casserole and bake in a 350° F oven for 40 minutes.

NUTRITION PER SERVING

		Calories:	249		
Carbohydrate:	6 g	Cholesterol:	126 mg	Potassium:	261 mg
Protein:	29 g	Fiber:	.6 g	Calcium:	134 mg
Total Fat:	12 g	Sodium:	424 mg	Iron:	4.8 mg

CHILI CON CARNE

(dairy-free, egg-free, gluten-free, sugar-free, yeast-free)   *Makes 4 servings*

When you serve a bean dish over rice, you create a protein that is equal to meat, poultry, or fish. In this instance, you can use a smaller amount of beef or add another can of kidney beans to stretch the recipe to feed more. Not expensive, but hearty and good!

INGREDIENTS
1 tablespoon olive oil
2 medium onions, finely diced
1 pound lean ground beef
2 teaspoons chili powder
1/2 teaspoon salt
1/2 teaspoon paprika
1/4 teaspoon Tabasco sauce
1 (16-ounce) can tomatoes
1 (6-ounce) can tomato paste
1 (20-ounce) can kidney beans
2 cups cooked enriched white rice

Heat oil in a large skillet over low heat. Add onions and sauté until limp. Add crumbled up bits of ground beef; break apart with a fork while browning. Sprinkle with chili powder, salt, paprika, and Tabasco sauce. Add tomatoes and tomato paste. Cover and simmer for 15 minutes. Add kidney beans and simmer 15 minutes longer. Serve over cooked rice.

NUTRITION PER SERVING
Calories: 498

Carbohydrate:	59 g	Cholesterol:	77 mg	Potassium:	1,170 mg
Protein:	35 g	Fiber:	2.6 g	Calcium:	91 mg
Total Fat:	13 g	Sodium:	868 mg	Iron:	7.4 mg

BEEF CHOP SUEY

(dairy-free, egg-free, gluten-free, sugar-free, yeast-free)   *Makes 3 servings*

For those who own an Oriental wok and enjoy the stir-fry method of cooking, the following recipe should be fun to try. The technique makes use of very little oil, but be sure to stir-fry throughout the cooking time. A large skillet can easily be substituted for the wok.

INGREDIENTS
½ pound beef flank steak
1 tablespoon corn oil
2 celery stalks, thinly sliced
1 cup sliced Chinese cabbage
1 large onion, thinly sliced
1 cup fresh bean sprouts
½ teaspoon salt
⅛ teaspoon pepper
¾ cup cold water
2 teaspoons cornstarch
1 cup hot cooked enriched white rice

Slice flank steak into thin pieces. (It is easiest to do if the steak is slightly frozen.) Rub the wok or a skillet with oil, coating well. Heat the wok very hot and sauté beef strips quickly, stir-frying continuously, about 2 minutes. Add celery, Chinese cabbage, onion, and bean sprouts; sauté 2 minutes more. Add salt, pepper, and ½ cup of the cold water. Cover and cook 7 minutes or until vegetables are soft. Combine cornstarch and ¼ cup of the water and mix into a thin paste. Add cornstarch mixture to the wok and mix; cook another 2 minutes, until liquid is thickened and clear. Serve over cooked rice.

NUTRITION PER SERVING

		Calories:	330		
Carbohydrate:	33 g	Cholesterol:	69 mg	Potassium:	533 mg
Protein:	27 g	Fiber:	8 g	Calcium:	57 mg
Total Fat:	8 g	Sodium:	826 mg	Iron:	4.3 mg

SWISS STEAK

(dairy-free, egg-free)   *Makes 8 servings*

The secret of making good Swiss steak is to braise it. That means, cook it slowly in liquid until the meat becomes very tender and well done. Browning the meat first sears in the juices—a step not to be missed with this cut of meat. Yeast-free dieters should not cook with wine—they can use tomato juice instead.

INGREDIENTS
2 pounds round steak, cut 1½ inches thick
1 garlic clove, finely chopped
¼ cup unbleached flour
¼ teaspoon paprika
⅛ teaspoon pepper
2 tablespoons olive oil
1 large onion, finely sliced
1 carrot, finely sliced
2 celery stalks, finely sliced
1 fresh dill sprig
½ teaspoon salt
2 tomatoes, chopped
¼ cup water
¼ cup dry red wine, such as burgundy

Rub steak with chopped garlic on both sides. Combine flour, paprika, and pepper. Pound flour mixture into the surface of the meat, using a meat mallet or heavy saucer. Heat oil in a large heavy skillet and sauté onion over medium heat until translucent; push aside. Brown meat in the skillet, turning to sear all sides. Lower heat and add carrot, celery, dill, salt, and tomatoes. Add water and wine. Cover tightly and cook over low heat for 2 hours, or until tender, adding additional boiling water if needed.

NUTRITION PER SERVING
Calories: 285

Carbohydrate:	7 g	Cholesterol:	103 mg	Potassium:	565 mg
Protein:	36 g	Fiber:	.4 g	Calcium:	31 mg
Total Fat:	5 g	Sodium:	221 mg	Iron:	4.6 mg

BEEF BOURGUIGNONNE

(dairy-free, egg-free, gluten-free, sugar-free) *Makes 8 servings*

This baked beef stew could be cooked over low heat on top of the range, but it tastes so much better when baked the French way—with heat coming at the pot from all sides. You cannot make too much, because it freezes and reheats superbly. Yeast-free dieters should omit the wine and mushrooms.

INGREDIENTS

2 pounds boned lean beef, cut in cubes
1 teaspoon garlic powder
1 teaspoon paprika
1/2 teaspoon salt
2 tablespoons olive oil
1 cup burgundy wine
12 tiny whole white onions, or 3 large sliced onions
2 beef bouillon cubes
2 cups boiling water
2 tablespoons tomato paste
1/2 teaspoon dried thyme
1/4 teaspoon pepper
2 bay leaves
6 carrots, scraped and cut into chunks
6 potatoes, peeled and quartered
1/2 pound fresh mushrooms, sliced

Season beef cubes with garlic powder and paprika. Place oil in a Dutch oven and heat on top of the range. Brown beef cubes lightly on all sides, turning them with a long wooden spoon. Pour wine over beef. Arrange onions around beef. Combine bouillon cubes and boiling water in a medium bowl, stir to dissolve and then mix in tomato paste, thyme, and pepper. Pour bouillon mixture over beef. Add bay leaves, carrots, potatoes, and mushrooms. Cover and place in a 350° F oven. Bake for 2 hours, or until meat is tender.

NUTRITION PER SERVING

		Calories:	392		
Carbohydrate:	25 g	Cholesterol:	104 mg	Potassium:	1,076 mg
Protein:	40 g	Fiber:	1.5 g	Calcium:	54 mg
Total Fat:	11 g	Sodium:	474 mg	Iron:	5.9 mg

CURRIED BEEF STEW

(dairy-free, egg-free, gluten-free, sugar-free, yeast-free)   *Makes 4 servings*

Here's a zesty pot of stew to consider for a weekend at home. With extra vegetables, it could be stretched to feed more.

INGREDIENTS
2 tablespoons olive oil
1 pound well-trimmed beef chuck, cut into small chunks
1 (16-ounce) can tomatoes
1 tablespoon chili powder
1 teaspoon curry powder
½ teaspoon salt
12 small white onions
4 carrots, scraped and cut into chunks
1 pound green beans, trimmed

Heat oil in a large heavy saucepan; sauté beef chunks over medium heat until nicely browned. Add tomatoes, chili powder, curry powder, salt, onions, and carrots. Cover, reduce heat to low, and simmer until beef is tender, about 1 to 1½ hours. Add whole trimmed green beans during the last ½ hour of cooking.

NUTRITION PER SERVING
Calories: 388

Carbohydrate:	13 g	Cholesterol:	71 mg	Potassium:	635 mg
Protein:	20 g	Fiber:	1.4 g	Calcium:	61 mg
Total Fat:	28 g	Sodium:	354 mg	Iron:	3.3 mg

BROILED CALF'S LIVER

(dairy-free, egg-free, gluten-free, sugar-free, yeast-free)   *Makes 4 servings*

The best way to cook liver is to broil it quickly and serve at once. Liver is an excellent source of iron, B vitamins, and protein. It is inexpensive, so you can plan to eat it at least once a week to save money while you boost your nutritional intake.

INGREDIENTS
4 slices calf's liver, about 1 pound
1 teaspoon olive oil
1/4 teaspoon salt
1/8 teaspoon pepper
1/8 teaspoon ground dried sage

Brush pieces of liver with olive oil. Sprinkle with salt, pepper, and sage. Place on a broiling pan about 5 inches from source of heat. Broil for 4 minutes, then turn and broil other side for 4 minutes more. Serve at once.

NUTRITION PER SERVING
Calories: 196

Carbohydrate:	3 g	Cholesterol:	340 mg	Potassium:	171 mg
Protein:	30 g	Fiber:	0 g	Calcium:	13 mg
Total Fat:	6 g	Sodium:	202 mg	Iron:	9.6 mg

BRAISED SHOULDER LAMB CHOPS

(*dairy-free, egg-free, gluten-free, sugar-free, yeast-free*)   *Makes 2 servings*

Shoulder lamb chops are not quite as tasty as the rib chops but they have less fat and are less expensive. When cooked as in this recipe, they are very tasty indeed!

INGREDIENTS
1 tablespoon olive oil
2 shoulder lamb chops, about ½-inch thick
1 large onion, thinly sliced
1 garlic clove, minced
1 cup sliced celery
1 green pepper, finely diced
½ cup tomato juice
1 bay leaf
½ teaspoon salt
¼ teaspoon pepper
¼ teaspoon dried basil

Heat oil in a large skillet. Add chops and cook over medium heat until lightly browned on both sides. Add onion, garlic, celery, and green pepper. Cover and cook over low heat for 15 minutes. Add tomato juice, bay leaf, salt, pepper, and basil. Cover and cook over low heat for 20 minutes more, or until lamb is tender.

NUTRITION PER SERVING
Calories: 326

Carbohydrate:	10 g	Cholesterol:	113 mg	Potassium:	809 mg
Protein:	31 g	Fiber:	1.2 g	Calcium:	57 mg
Total Fat:	17 g	Sodium:	817 mg	Iron:	2.9 mg

BAKED EGGS IN SPINACH NESTS

(*dairy-free, sugar-free*)   *Makes 4 servings*

*When you are rummaging for meal possibilities with an almost empty larder,
gather some eggs, frozen spinach, and some English muffins to make this
delicious and easy baked dish.*

INGREDIENTS
2 English muffins, split in halves
1 (10-ounce) package frozen chopped spinach, cooked and drained
1/4 teaspoon nutmeg
1/4 teaspoon onion powder
1/8 teaspoon pepper
4 eggs
Paprika to garnish

Arrange muffin halves on a cookie sheet. Add to cooked spinach the
nutmeg, onion powder, and pepper; mix well. Spoon 1/4 of the spinach onto
each muffin half, making an indented "nest" in the center of each mound
with the back of a large spoon. Break 1 egg into each spinach nest. Top
each with a dash of paprika. Bake at 350° F for 15 minutes, or until eggs are
of desired firmness. Serve at once.

NUTRITION PER SERVING

				Calories:	160		
Carbohydrate:	16 g	Cholesterol:	274 mg	Potassium:	384 mg
Protein:	16 g	Fiber:	.5 g	Calcium:	133 mg
Total Fat:	7 g	Sodium:	220 mg	Iron:	3.6 mg

SPINACH-CHEESE SOUFFLÉ

(gluten-free, sugar-free, yeast-free)   *Makes 2 servings*

Spinach is high in beta-carotene, tucked into salads or cooked as below. Don't forget the nutmeg! It gives spinach just the kick of flavor that will make this one of your favorite last-minute meals.

INGREDIENTS
1 (10-ounce) package frozen chopped spinach
1/2 cup lowfat cottage cheese
2 eggs, separated
1/4 teaspoon salt
1/4 teaspoon dried dill
1/4 teaspoon ground nutmeg

Cook spinach according to package in a small amount of water and drain well. Combine cooked spinach, cottage cheese, egg yolks, salt, dill, and nutmeg in a medium bowl. Beat egg whites in a small bowl until stiff peaks form. Fold gently into the spinach mixture. Pour into a nonstick baking dish. Bake in a 350° F oven for 20 minutes, or until firm.

NUTRITION PER SERVING
Calories: 156

Carbohydrate:	8 g	Cholesterol:	276 mg	Potassium:	696 mg
Protein:	24 g	Fiber:	1.1 g	Calcium:	231 mg
Total Fat:	7 g	Sodium:	417 mg	Iron:	5 mg

SPINACH FRITTATA

(gluten-free, sugar-free)   *Makes 6 servings*

How do you make an impromptu light supper when you've nothing but eggs,
some mushrooms, and a package of frozen spinach in the larder? Here's one way
to do it nicely! Yeast-free dieters should omit the mushrooms.

INGREDIENTS

1 (10-ounce) package frozen chopped spinach
1/2 pound fresh mushrooms, sliced
1 small onion, finely diced
2 tablespoons corn oil margarine
6 eggs
1/2 teaspoon salt
1/8 teaspoon pepper
2 tablespoons grated Parmesan cheese

Cook spinach according to package and drain well. Sauté mushrooms and
onion in margarine in a large ovenproof skillet over medium heat. Beat
eggs, salt, and pepper together in a medium bowl; stir in drained spinach
and mix well. Pour mixture over mushrooms and onions in the skillet. Cook
over medium heat until eggs are set. Sprinkle with Parmesan cheese and
run under the broiler until cheese melts and the top is lightly browned. Cut
into wedges and serve at once.

NUTRITION PER SERVING

		Calories:	136		
Carbohydrate:	4 g	Cholesterol:	275 mg	Potassium:	322 mg
Protein:	15 g	Fiber:	.5 g	Calcium:	116 mg
Total Fat:	10 g	Sodium:	331 mg	Iron:	2.5 mg

15

NUTRITIOUS NO-COOK MEALS

THERE ARE MOMENTS WHEN YOU NEED TO take the easy way out. If you market with this in mind, you will always be able to open a few items and combine them into a well-balanced meal.

For instance, keep a fresh supply of low-fat cottage cheese, nonfat yogurt, and salad vegetables in the refrigerator. Among those vegetables should be lettuce, tomatoes, green peppers, carrots, and celery. Recipes in this section will demonstrate that such a larder can produce a well-balanced meal in minutes.

While emphasizing freshness and variety in your food supply, you do need a backup of such canned goods as water-packed tuna, sardines, salmon, crabmeat, garbanzo beans, red kidney beans, white navy beans, sliced beets, and artichoke hearts, to name a few.

Go for the new "light" mayonnaise-type dressing to use for salad mixtures. To further reduce fat content, combine it half and half with nonfat yogurt. Stir in a sprinkling of dill or parsley to add more flavor to tuna and cold diced chicken.

Whenever you opt for a sandwich, be sure to use whole-grain bread and tuck in some vegetables. Lettuce and tomato are a natural, but sprouts, cucumber, or zucchini slices can also be effective. Think of variety, even when it's a no-cook meal!

ANTIPASTO

(dairy-free, egg-free, gluten-free)   *Makes 4 servings*

There are times when an interesting main course can be created hastily from an assortment of cans and jars. You can do it only if you remember to keep such a backup stock in your pantry shelf. Pickled items usually have sugar and vinegar (a no-no for yeast avoiders).

INGREDIENTS
1 (7-ounce) can water-packed tuna fish
1 (16-ounce) jar pickled beets and onions

184

1 (6-ounce) jar pickled artichoke hearts
1 (4³/₄-ounce) can whole sardines in oil
1 (4¹/₄-ounce) can eggplant caponata
1 cup whole cherry tomatoes
1 cucumber, sliced thin
Lettuce leaves

Open all cans and jars; drain well. Prepare the tomatoes and cucumber. Arrange each ingredient on a lettuce cup and set on a suitable platter or tray. Each person then serves himself some of each dish.

NUTRITION PER SERVING

		Calories:	159		
Carbohydrate:	14 g	Cholesterol:	65 mg	Potassium:	633 mg
Protein:	20 g	Fiber:	1.4 g	Calcium:	139 mg
Total Fat:	2 g	Sodium:	400 mg	Iron:	2.7 mg

COTTAGE CHEESE–VEGETABLE SALAD

(egg-free, gluten-free, sugar-free, yeast-free)   *Makes 4 servings*

Here's a no-cook salad meal that is chock-full of vitamins, minerals, and protein. This makes a good lunch or light supper.

INGREDIENTS
1 large cucumber, peeled and diced
4 radishes, sliced
1 green pepper, diced
2 celery stalks, thinly sliced
1 large tomato, cut into wedges
2 cups low-fat cottage cheese
¹/₂ cup plain nonfat yogurt
2 tablespoons chopped dried chives

Place all cut vegetables into a salad bowl. Add cottage cheese; stir lightly until all is mixed through. Combine the yogurt and chives. Serve with yogurt-chive mixture as a dressing.

NUTRITION PER SERVING

		Calories:	117		
Carbohydrate:	9 g	Cholesterol:	5 mg	Potassium:	388 mg
Protein:	16 g	Fiber:	.6 g	Calcium:	144 mg
Total Fat:	1 g	Sodium:	30 mg	Iron:	.7 mg

STUFFED TOMATO SURPRISE

(*egg-free, gluten-free, sugar-free, yeast-free*)   *Makes 1 serving*

If you remember to keep a container of low-fat cottage cheese in your refrigerator, you will always have a high-protein meal possibility. Here it is stuffed into a tomato.

INGREDIENTS
1 large tomato
Salad greens
1/2 green pepper, finely diced
1 celery stalk, finely diced
1 carrot, scraped and grated
1 tablespoon chopped dried chives
1/2 cup low-fat cottage cheese
1 tablespoon plain nonfat yogurt
1 orange, peeled and sliced

Wash tomato and cut into wedges without cutting all the way through the bottom. Spread tomato open. Place tomato on a bed of salad greens. Combine green pepper, celery, carrot, chives, and cottage cheese in a small bowl. Mound this on top of spread tomato wedges. Top with yogurt. Arrange sliced oranges alongside tomato.

NUTRITION PER SERVING

		Calories:	237		
Carbohydrate:	39 g	Cholesterol:	6 mg	Potassium:	1,266 mg
Protein:	21 g	Fiber:	3 g	Calcium:	262 mg
Total Fat:	1 g	Sodium:	97 mg	Iron:	2.6 mg

CHICKEN WALDORF SALAD

(*dairy-free, gluten-free, sugar-free*)   *Makes 3 servings*

So you have a bit of left-over chicken or turkey on hand and want to extend it into a cold salad? If you have an apple, some celery, walnuts, and raisins you can make this delightful concoction. Mmmm good! Because mayonnaise contains vinegar, yeast-free dieters should use yogurt instead.

INGREDIENTS
1 cup diced cooked chicken
1 apple with peel, cored and diced

1 celery stalk, diced
¼ cup seedless raisins
¼ cup walnut halves
2 tablespoons light mayonnaise
¼ teaspoon dried tarragon

Combine all the ingredients in a medium bowl; mix well. Chill until ready to serve.

NUTRITION PER SERVING
Calories: 110

Carbohydrate:	17 g	Cholesterol:	44 mg	Potassium:	269 mg
Protein:	7 g	Fiber:	.6 g	Calcium:	20 mg
Total Fat:	2 g	Sodium:	46 mg	Iron:	1.1 mg

AVOCADO-CRABMEAT SALAD

(egg-free, gluten-free, sugar-free, yeast-free)   *Makes 4 servings*

Choose avocados that are slightly soft to the touch. Or leave them at room temperature until they are ripe; then refrigerate until ready to use.

INGREDIENTS
2 (7½-ounce) cans Alaska king crabmeat
Salad greens
1 (16-ounce) can unsweetened grapefruit sections, drained
2 ripe avocados, peeled and pitted
1 tablespoon lemon juice
2 tablespoons plain nonfat yogurt
5 tablespoons low-fat cottage cheese
¼ teaspoon dried dill

Arrange crabmeat on salad greens on a platter. Garnish with grapefruit sections. Slice avocados and arrange on the platter; drizzle lemon juice over avocados. Combine yogurt, cottage cheese, and dill in a small bowl and use as a dressing for the salad.

NUTRITION PER SERVING
Calories: 295

Carbohydrate:	15 g	Cholesterol:	70 mg	Potassium:	879 mg
Protein:	18 g	Fiber:	1.8 g	Calcium:	85 mg
Total Fat:	20 g	Sodium:	681 mg	Iron:	1.7 mg

TUNA AND WHITE BEAN SALAD

(*dairy-free, egg-free, gluten-free, sugar-free*)   *Makes 2 servings*

Here's a nutritious no-cook meal that is good for lunch or dinner. Delicious tucked into pita bread! Yeast-free dieters can omit the vinegar.

INGREDIENTS
1 (7-ounce) can water-packed tuna fish, drained
1 (16-ounce) can white Italian beans, drained
1 small onion, thinly sliced
1 garlic clove, minced
2 tablespoons olive oil
1 tablespoon tarragon vinegar
1 teaspoon dried basil

Flake tuna into a medium bowl. Add white beans. Add onion, garlic, oil, vinegar, and basil. Toss well. Serve on lettuce or as a sandwich, if desired.

NUTRITION PER SERVING

		Calories:	357		
Carbohydrate:	22 g	Cholesterol:	52 mg	Potassium:	699 mg
Protein:	35 g	Fiber:	1.5 g	Calcium:	68 mg
Total Fat:	14 g	Sodium:	50 mg	Iron:	4.7 mg

TUNA-VEGETABLE SALAD

(*egg-free, gluten-free, sugar-free, yeast-free*)   *Makes 3 servings*

Tuna contains Omega-3 fatty acids, which reduce LDL in the bloodsteam. Stir some vegetables into your tuna salad mixture to make it stretch further and have better balanced nutrition. This is good on a bed of greens or stuffed into pita bread or other sandwich makings.

INGREDIENTS
1 (7-ounce) can water-packed tuna fish, drained
1 celery stalk, finely diced
1 carrot, scraped and grated
1/4 cup finely diced red onion
1/4 cup plain nonfat yogurt
1/4 teaspoon dried tarragon

Flake tuna into a medium bowl with a fork. Add celery, carrot, onion, yogurt, and tarragon; mix well. Makes 3 servings

NUTRITION PER SERVING

Calories: 111

Carbohydrate:	6 g	Cholesterol:	34 mg	Potassium:	382 mg
Protein:	20 g	Fiber:	.4 g	Calcium:	67 mg
Total Fat:	.3 g	Sodium:	56 mg	Iron:	1.4 mg

FISH SALAD

(egg-free, gluten-free, sugar-free, yeast-free)   *Makes 2 servings*

Whenever you have some fish left over, refrigerate it and turn it into a fish salad for the next day's lunch or dinner. This makes a good platter or sandwich.

INGREDIENTS

1 cup flaked cooked fish
1 celery stalk, finely diced
2 tablespoons diced red onion
$^1/_2$ teaspoon dried dill
$^1/_4$ teaspoon salt
$^1/_8$ teaspoon pepper
2 tablespoons plain nonfat yogurt
1 teaspoon pickle relish (optional)
Salad greens

Combine flaked fish, celery, onion, dill, salt, pepper, yogurt, and relish in a medium bowl; mix well. Line a plate with salad greens. Place fish mixture in a mound on the greens.

NUTRITION PER SERVING

Calories: 134

Carbohydrate:	4 g	Cholesterol:	35 mg	Potassium:	526 mg
Protein:	18 g	Fiber:	.3 g	Calcium:	73 mg
Total Fat:	4 g	Sodium:	429 mg	Iron:	1.3 mg

SARDINE SALAD

(dairy-free, gluten-free, sugar-free, yeast-free)   *Makes 2 servings*

Sardines are high in calcium and convenient to keep on the pantry shelf. Here's a nice way to turn them into a salad. Mayonnaise has vinegar so yeast-free dieters should use yogurt instead.

INGREDIENTS
1 (8-ounce) can sardines packed in tomato sauce, with bones
1 tablespoon lemon juice
1 hard-cooked egg, chopped
1 tablespoon light mayonnaise
Shredded lettuce
Carrot sticks
Tomato wedges

Mash sardines with lemon juice in a medium bowl. Add chopped egg; stir in mayonnaise. Place shredded lettuce on a plate and mound sardine mixture on top. Garnish with carrot sticks and tomato wedges.

NUTRITION PER SERVING
Calories: 318

Carbohydrate:	9 g	Cholesterol:	274 mg	Potassium:	1,058 mg
Protein:	31 g	Fiber:	.9 g	Calcium:	552 mg
Total Fat:	16 g	Sodium:	995 mg	Iron:	4.8 mg

16

VITAL VEGETABLES

WHEN YOU ARE CHOOSING VEGETABLES, think of the food chain that brings them to your table. Try to select those vegetables that have been the least handled and seasoned on their way to you. This puts fresh vegetables first, frozen vegetables second, and canned vegetables last.

The best way to cook fresh vegetables is to steam them. This is easy to do if you have a perforated rack that will fit into a saucepan or skillet. Just fill the bottom with water, place the vegetables on the perforated rack set over the water, cover, bring the water to a boil, and steam until tender.

If you choose to cook the vegetables in water, use as little water as possible to get the job done. Nutrients will leach out into the water—if you can add this cooking liquid to soup it is a worthwhile saving.

Avoid sauces and globs of butter to cut down on fat intake that is unnecessary and not a natural component of vegetables. Avoid any frozen vegetables that have been sauced and salted. Vegetables have a wonderful flavor when cooked right—overcooking destroys valuable nutrients.

Sometimes, as with asparagus, broccoli, and green beans, crispness is desired. Washed spinach should be cooked in the water that clings to it only until wilted. Artichokes need to be cooked until you can easily scrape the goodies off the leaves. Potatoes should be fork tender, whether baked or boiled. Broaden your vegetable horizons with these recipes!

BAKED ACORN SQUASH

(dairy-free, egg-free, gluten-free, sugar-free, yeast-free)   *Makes 2 servings*

There are two kinds of squash—summer squash, such as zucchini and yellow crookneck, and winter squash, such as acorn and butternut. The hardy winter squash may be stored at cool temperature for many months, if you have such a place. Otherwise, the refrigerator is the best way to store it. You'll find that acorn squash has the flavor of a nutty sweet potato!

INGREDIENTS
1 acorn squash
1 teaspoon corn oil margarine
$1/4$ teaspoon nutmeg
$1/4$ teaspoon cinnamon

Cut acorn squash in half lengthwise. Scoop out seeds and discard. Place squash, cut side up, in a baking pan. Fill squash cavities with dots of margarine and sprinkle with nutmeg and cinnamon. Bake in a 350° F oven for 25 minutes, or until fork tender.

NUTRITION PER SERVING
Calories: 80

Carbohydrate:	16 g	Cholesterol:	0 mg	Potassium:	473 mg
Protein:	2 g	Fiber:	1.8 g	Calcium:	29 mg
Total Fat:	2 g	Sodium:	23 mg	Iron:	.8 mg

GREEN BEANS AMANDINE

(dairy-free, egg-free, gluten-free, yeast-free)   *Makes 4 servings*

Of course, green beans are delicious when fresh and steamed to semicrispness. To dress them up even more, use this trick with almonds.

INGREDIENTS
1 pound fresh green beans, or 1 (10-ounce) package frozen
1 teaspoon corn oil margarine
$1/2$ teaspoon chopped parsley
2 tablespoons sliced almonds

Trim ends of green beans and rinse beans well. Place beans in a steamer basket over boiling water, or in a heavy pot with a small amount of water.

Cook until just limp, about 5 minutes. Drain and put into a medium bowl. Toss with margarine and parsley. Top with sliced almonds and serve hot.

NUTRITION PER SERVING

		Calories:	47		
Carbohydrate:	4 g	Cholesterol:	0 mg	Potassium:	128 mg
Protein:	2 g	Fiber:	.8 g	Calcium:	42 mg
Total Fat:	3 g	Sodium:	14 mg	Iron:	.6 mg

HERBED GREEN BEANS AND ONIONS

(dairy-free, egg-free, gluten-free, sugar-free, yeast-free)   *Makes 4 servings*

There are times when you want to dress up steamed green beans to make them fancy enough for company fare. Those are the times when your herb shelf comes to the rescue!

INGREDIENTS
¾ pound fresh green beans, or 1 (10-ounce) package frozen
1 medium onion, thinly sliced
1 tablespoon corn oil margarine
1 teaspoon dried parsley
1 teaspoon dried rosemary

Wash and trim fresh green beans. Steam fresh or frozen beans over hot water or cook in a small amount of water until tender, about 10 minutes. Sauté onion in margarine in a small nonstick skillet over medium heat, until onion is limp. Add parsley and rosemary. Drain beans and put in medium bowl. Pour onion mixture over beans, toss, and serve.

NUTRITION PER SERVING

		Calories:	45		
Carbohydrate:	5 g	Cholesterol:	0 mg	Potassium:	120 mg
Protein:	1 g	Fiber:	.7 g	Calcium:	37 mg
Total Fat:	2 g	Sodium:	38 mg	Iron:	.5 mg

GREEN BEANS OREGANO

(dairy-free, egg-free, gluten-free, sugar-free, yeast-free)   *Makes 6 servings*

Maybe you like your green beans just as they come from the fields and maybe you prefer a bit of dressing up. Here's the way to add some flair to an ordinary garden vegetable.

INGREDIENTS

1 pound fresh green beans, stemmed and sliced
3 tomatoes, cut in small wedges
1 small onion, thinly sliced
1/2 teaspoon salt
1/8 teaspoon pepper
1/4 teaspoon oregano

Place green beans in a medium size, heavy saucepan. Add 1 inch of water. Add tomato wedges, onion, salt, pepper, and oregano. Simmer over medium heat until beans are tender, about 15 minutes. Remove with a slotted spoon and serve.

NUTRITION PER SERVING

		Calories:	31		
Carbohydrate:	7 g	Cholesterol:	0 mg	Potassium:	260 mg
Protein:	1 g	Fiber:	1 g	Calcium:	43 mg
Total Fat:	trace	Sodium:	183 mg	Iron:	.7 mg

BROCCOLI WITH PARSLEY SAUCE

(dairy-free, egg-free, gluten-free, sugar-free, yeast-free)   *Makes 4 servings*

If the stalks of broccoli are thick and tough, scrape the outer layer off with a paring knife. Cook only until tender, but still green. Dreadful things are done to broccoli by overcooking it into gray-green limpness!

INGREDIENTS

1 bunch broccoli, about 1 pound
2 tablespoons corn oil margarine
2 tablespoons chopped fresh parsley
1 lemon, cut in wedges

Wash broccoli under cold water. Trim ends. Pare if necessary. Cut lengthwise into halves or quarters if stems are very thick. Place broccoli into a large skillet or saucepan. Add 1 inch of water. Cook over medium heat until just tender, about 10 minutes. Melt margarine in a small saucepan; stir in parsley. Place cooked broccoli on a warm platter, pour sauce over all and serve with lemon wedges.

NUTRITION PER SERVING

		Calories:	88		
Carbohydrate:	7 g	Cholesterol:	0 mg	Potassium:	400 mg
Protein:	5 g	Fiber:	2 g	Calcium:	128 mg
Total Fat:	6 g	Sodium:	83 mg	Iron:	1.2 mg

BRUSSELS SPROUTS AND TOMATOES

(dairy-free, egg-free, gluten-free, sugar-free, yeast-free)   *Makes 4 servings*

Use fresh Brussels sprouts when they are in season. Cook until tender but not mushy. You'll love the delicate cabbage flavor!

INGREDIENTS
1 pint fresh Brussels sprouts
2 tomatoes, cut in thin wedges
1/2 cup water
1/2 teaspoon salt
1/8 teaspoon pepper
1 teaspoon lemon juice
1 tablespoon chopped fresh parsley

Wash Brussels sprouts thoroughly, trim stems, and cut in half lengthwise. Place Brussels sprouts in a medium saucepan. Add tomatoes, water, salt, pepper, lemon juice, and parsley. Cover tightly and cook over medium heat 10 to 15 minutes until tender.

NUTRITION PER SERVING

		Calories:	40		
Carbohydrate:	8 g	Cholesterol:	0 mg	Potassium:	185 mg
Protein:	4 g	Fiber:	.8 g	Calcium:	18 mg
Total Fat:	.5 g	Sodium:	138 mg	Iron:	.6 mg

SWEET-AND-SOUR RED CABBAGE

(dairy-free, egg-free, gluten-free) *Makes 6 servings*

Red cabbage is an excellent vegetable to keep in the crisper of the refrigerator to add to green salads. If the cabbage gets a bit wilted, cook it this sweet-and-sour way and serve it as a hot vegetable. Yeast-free dieters should omit the sugar and vinegar. Hypoglycemics should omit the sugar.

INGREDIENTS
1 medium head red cabbage, shredded
1 cup water
1 teaspoon brown sugar
1 tablespoon tarragon vinegar
2 whole cloves
$\frac{1}{2}$ teaspoon ground ginger
$\frac{1}{2}$ teaspoon salt
$\frac{1}{4}$ teaspoon pepper

Place cabbage in a large deep saucepan. Add water, sugar, vinegar, cloves, ginger, salt, and pepper. Cover and simmer 30 minutes over low heat, stirring occasionally, or until cabbage is tender.

NUTRITION PER SERVING

		Calories:	13		
Carbohydrate:	3 g	Cholesterol:	0 mg	Potassium:	99 mg
Protein:	.5 g	Fiber:	.3 g	Calcium:	16 mg
Total Fat:	trace	Sodium:	186 mg	Iron:	.3 mg

PINEAPPLE COLESLAW WITH YOGURT DRESSING

(egg-free, gluten-free)   *Makes 6 servings*

This slaw is stripped of fat and sugar but not of taste! Yeast-free dieters should omit the vinegar and honey. Hypoglycemics should omit the honey.

INGREDIENTS
3/4 cup plain nonfat yogurt
2 teaspoons red wine vinegar
2 teaspoons honey
1 tablespoon grated onion
1/8 teaspoon pepper
1/4 teaspoon celery seed
1/8 teaspoon dry mustard
2 cups shredded white cabbage
1/2 cup grated carrots
1/2 cup unsweetened crushed pineapple, drained

Combine yogurt, vinegar, honey, onion, pepper, celery seed, and dry mustard in a small bowl; mix well. Combine cabbage, carrots, and pineapple in a large bowl. Add yogurt mixture to the cabbage and toss well. Chill.

NUTRITION PER SERVING

		Calories:	40		
Carbohydrate:	9 g	Cholesterol:	.5 mg	Potassium:	182 mg
Protein:	2 g	Fiber:	.4 g	Calcium:	74 mg
Total Fat:	trace	Sodium:	9 mg	Iron:	.3 mg

PICKLED VEGETABLE SALAD

(dairy-free, egg-free, gluten-free)   *Makes 8 servings*

This is more than a coleslaw and will keep longer because the vinegar dressing pickles the ingredients as the days go by. It is best when marinated in the dressing for at least 1 day. Substitute 2 tablespoons lemon juice if you are on a yeast-free diet.

INGREDIENTS
1 small head cabbage, thinly sliced
4 carrots, scraped and thinly sliced
2 cucumbers, peeled and thinly sliced
1 Bermuda onion, thinly sliced
1 green pepper, diced
1/2 cup salad oil
1/2 cup tarragon vinegar
1/2 cup water
1/2 teaspoon salt
1/2 teaspoon celery seed

Place all vegetables into a large deep bowl. Combine oil, vinegar, water, salt, and celery seed in a small bowl. Pour dressing over vegetables and mix well. Cover tightly and store in the refrigerator for at least 1 day before using.

NUTRITION PER SERVING

Calories: 62

Carbohydrate:	9 g	Cholesterol:	0 mg	Potassium:	284 mg
Protein:	1 g	Fiber:	1.4 g	Calcium:	40 mg
Total Fat:	3 g	Sodium:	161 mg	Iron:	.8 mg

CARROTS ROSEMARY

(dairy-free, egg-free, gluten-free, sugar-free, yeast-free)   *Makes 6 servings*

When you need a simple and yet elegant way to present freshly cooked carrots, make a bouillon sauce and sprinkle with a bit of herbs. For a change of pace, instead of slicing into rounds, slice the carrots into thin 3-inch sticks.

INGREDIENTS
4 large or 8 small carrots, scraped and sliced
1/2 cup water
1 bouillon cube
1 teaspoon corn oil margarine
1 teaspoon chopped fresh parsley
1/2 teaspoon dried rosemary
1/8 teaspoon salt
Dash of pepper

Place prepared carrots in a medium-size, heavy saucepan with the water and bouillon cube. Cover and cook over medium heat for 10 minutes, or until carrots are tender. Add margarine, parsley, rosemary, salt, and pepper. Mix well. Cook for 2 minutes more. Serve hot.

NUTRITION PER SERVING
Calories: 26

Carbohydrate:	5 g	Cholesterol:	.1 mg	Potassium:	166 mg
Protein:	.8 g	Fiber:	.4 g	Calcium:	19 mg
Total Fat:	.7 g	Sodium:	235 mg	Iron:	.3 mg

CARROTS VERONIQUE

(dairy-free, egg-free, gluten-free)   *Makes 6 servings*

There's nothing better for you than a raw scraped carrot, no fuss, no muss. But there are times when you want to show off a bit with your vegetable presentations. Here's one way to do it! Yeast-free dieters may omit the wine.

INGREDIENTS
4 large or 8 small carrots
1 teaspoon corn oil margarine
1 tablespoon lemon juice
1 tablespoon white wine
½ cup seedless green grapes

Scrape and slice the carrots. Place carrots in a medium-size, heavy saucepan with a small amount of water. Cover and cook over medium heat for 10 minutes, or until tender. Drain, keep in pan, and toss with margarine. Add lemon juice and white wine; stir well. Add grapes and simmer over low heat for 2 minutes more. Serve hot.

NUTRITION PER SERVING
Calories: 42

Carbohydrate:	8 g	Cholesterol:	0 mg	Potassium:	201 mg
Protein:	.7 g	Fiber:	.7 g	Calcium:	21 mg
Total Fat:	.7 g	Sodium:	31 mg	Iron:	.4 mg

CARROT STRIPS

(dairy-free, egg-free, gluten-free, sugar-free, yeast-free)   *Makes 2 servings*

Carrots are chock-full of beta-carotene, considered to be a cancer deterrent. Although this dark yellow vegetable is best eaten raw, here's a way to cook them to preserve their nutrients.

INGREDIENTS
2 large carrots, cut lengthwise into 4-inch strips
1 teaspoon chopped parsley
⅛ teaspoon tarragon
¼ cup water
1 teaspoon lemon juice

Place carrot strips, parsley, tarragon, and water in a medium-size saucepan; cover and simmer over low heat until carrots are tender, about 15 minutes, adding a little more water if necessary. Drain. Add lemon juice.

NUTRITION PER SERVING

		Calories:	30		
Carbohydrate:	7 g	Cholesterol:	0 mg	Potassium:	253 mg
Protein:	1 g	Fiber:	.7 g	Calcium:	28 mg
Total Fat:	trace	Sodium:	34 mg	Iron:	.5 mg

CAULIFLOWER AND TOMATOES PARMESAN

(egg-free, gluten-free, sugar-free, yeast-free)   *Makes 8 servings*

Wash cauliflower thoroughly to dislodge any possible hiding mites. Trim away any bruised areas. Then cook carefully, removing from heat when fork tender. Cooking too long will cause the cauliflower to fall apart. Dairy-free dieters can omit the Parmesan cheese.

INGREDIENTS
1 large head cauliflower
1 onion, diced
2 tablespoons chopped parsley
1 garlic clove, minced
1 (16-ounce) can stewed tomatoes
1/2 teaspoon salt
1/4 teaspoon pepper
1/4 teaspoon dried oregano
1/4 cup grated Parmesan cheese

Wash cauliflower thoroughly. Trim excess leaves and stem. Place cauliflower, head up, in a large, heavy saucepan. Add remaining ingredients to the saucepan, around the cauliflower. Cover and cook over low heat for 20 minutes, or until cauliflower is fork tender. Serve whole with the sauce.

NUTRITION PER SERVING

		Calories:	46		
Carbohydrate:	6 g	Cholesterol:	2 mg	Potassium:	288 mg
Protein:	4 g	Fiber:	10 g	Calcium:	65 mg
Total Fat:	1 g	Sodium:	242 mg	Iron:	.9 mg

PICKLED CUCUMBERS

(*dairy-free, egg-free, gluten-free*)   *Makes 6 servings*

*You may use regular onions for this, but the sweet Bermudas taste best if you can
find them in your market. Run the tines of a fork down the sides of the peeled
cucumbers for a slightly ruffled-looking edge when sliced! Yeast-dieters may
substitute 2 tablespoons lemon juice for the vinegar.*

INGREDIENTS
2 large cucumbers, peeled and thinly sliced
1 large onion, thinly sliced
1/4 cup red wine vinegar
2 tablespoons salad oil
1/4 teaspoon salt
1/8 teaspoon pepper

Place cucumbers and onion in a small deep bowl. Combine vinegar, oil,
salt, and pepper. Pour dressing over all and let marinate for several hours
before serving.

NUTRITION PER SERVING
Calories: 46

Carbohydrate:	2 g	Cholesterol:	0 mg	Potassium:	55 mg
Protein:	.2 g	Fiber:	.2 g	Calcium:	9 mg
Total Fat:	4 g	Sodium:	91 mg	Iron:	.3 mg

EGGPLANT PARMESAN

(egg-free, gluten-free, sugar-free, yeast-free)   *Makes 6 servings*

This eggplant recipe skips the usual advice to salt eggplant slices heavily and drain excess liquid before starting. You don't need that extra salt and making it this way works just fine.

INGREDIENTS

1 eggplant, peeled and sliced thin
2 cups tomato juice
2 tablespoons tomato paste
1/2 teaspoon salt
1/2 teaspoon oregano
1/4 teaspoon pepper
1/2 pound sliced low-fat mozzarella cheese
1/2 cup grated Parmesan cheese

Arrange several eggplant slices side-by-side in an 8 × 12-inch flat baking dish. Combine tomato juice, tomato paste, salt, oregano, and pepper in a medium bowl. Spoon some of the tomato sauce over the eggplant. Cover with thin slices of mozzarella cheese. Sprinkle lightly with Parmesan cheese. Repeat layers of eggplant, sauce, and cheese, making at least 2 layers, ending with cheese. Bake in a 350° F oven for 35 to 40 minutes, or until eggplant is fork tender.

NUTRITION PER SERVING

		Calories:	184		
Carbohydrate:	7 g	Cholesterol:	21 mg	Potassium:	320 mg
Protein:	13 g	Fiber:	.6 g	Calcium:	345 mg
Total Fat:	12 g	Sodium:	402 mg	Iron:	1.2 mg

BRAISED BELGIAN ENDIVES

(dairy-free, egg-free, gluten-free, sugar-free, yeast-free)   *Makes 4 servings*

Sometimes the most elegant side vegetables are quite simple to prepare. Belgian endives are usually served crisp leaved in a salad. In Belgium they are braised and served as a hot vegetable!

INGREDIENTS
4 Belgian endives
1 tablespoon corn oil margarine
1/4 teaspoon salt
1/4 cup water
1 tablespoon lemon juice
Pepper to taste

Wash endives under cold water; shake dry. Melt the margarine in a large skillet. Place endives in it. Add salt, water, and lemon juice. Cover the skillet tightly and cook over very low heat for about 10 minutes. Turn the endives and allow to cook for about 10 minutes longer. When endives are tender, remove the lid and allow the juices to cook down. Sprinkle with pepper.

NUTRITION PER SERVING

		Calories:	31		
Carbohydrate:	1 g	Cholesterol:	0 mg	Potassium:	79 mg
Protein:	.5 g	Fiber:	.2 g	Calcium:	20 mg
Total Fat:	2 g	Sodium:	170 mg	Iron:	.4 mg

SPINACH-ORANGE SALAD BOWL

(*dairy-free, egg-free, gluten-free, sugar-free, yeast-free*) *Makes 4 servings*

When planning to make a fresh spinach salad, be sure that the spinach leaves are crisp and clean. Rinse several times in cold water, then place in a wrapping of paper towels and refrigerate for several hours until crisp.

INGREDIENTS
2 tablespoons lemon juice
1/4 cup orange juice
1 tablespoon corn oil
1/4 teaspoon paprika
1/4 teaspoon celery salt
1/2 teaspoon garlic powder
Dash of pepper
4 cups torn fresh spinach leaves
4 sliced radishes
1 orange, peeled and cut into bite-size pieces

In a jar or blender, combine lemon juice, orange juice, oil, paprika, celery salt, garlic powder, and pepper. Mix thoroughly. Arrange spinach, radishes, and orange pieces in a salad bowl. Pour dressing over salad and toss lightly.

NUTRITION PER SERVING

		Calories:	70		
Carbohydrate:	8 g	Cholesterol:	0 mg	Potassium:	380 mg
Protein:	2 g	Fiber:	.5 g	Calcium:	68 mg
Total Fat:	3 g	Sodium:	40 mg	Iron:	1.9 mg

SPINACH SALAD

(dairy-free, egg-free, gluten-free, sugar-free)   *Makes 8 servings*

Garlic and onion can give spinach just the zest it needs! Yeast-free dieters may use 2 tablespoons lemon juice instead of the vinegar.

INGREDIENTS
1 pound fresh spinach
1 garlic clove
1/2 small red onion, thinly sliced
1/4 cup tomato juice
2 tablespoons olive oil
3 tablespoons red wine vinegar
1/2 teaspoon dry mustard
1/8 teaspoon pepper

Wash spinach several times, until water runs clear. Trim stems. Rub salad bowl with cut garlic clove; discard remaining garlic. Put spinach in the bowl. Add onion. Combine tomato juice, oil, vinegar, mustard, and pepper; pour over spinach. Toss well and serve.

NUTRITION PER SERVING

		Calories:	45		
Carbohydrate:	3 g	Cholesterol:	0 mg	Potassium:	209 mg
Protein:	2 g	Fiber:	.4 g	Calcium:	44 mg
Total Fat:	3.5 g	Sodium:	52 mg	Iron:	1.2 mg

CREAMED SPINACH

(egg-free, gluten-free, sugar-free, yeast-free)   *Makes 4 servings*

Here's a way to get the fat out of creamed spinach. Be careful not to cook the yogurt because it may curdle. Dairy-free dieters should omit the yogurt and use this method for cooking nutrient-rich spinach.

INGREDIENTS
1 pound fresh spinach
1 small onion, grated
1/4 teaspoon nutmeg
1/8 teaspoon pepper
1/2 cup plain nonfat yogurt

Wash spinach leaves and trim off roots and stems. Place in a large skillet with a small amount of water. Add onion, nutmeg, and pepper. Cook, covered, over low heat, until tender, about 5 minutes. Drain well. Toss with yogurt and serve.

NUTRITION PER SERVING

		Calories:	35		
Carbohydrate:	5 g	Cholesterol:	.5 mg	Potassium:	348 mg
Protein:	4 g	Fiber:	.4 g	Calcium:	110 mg
Total Fat:	trace	Sodium:	40 mg	Iron:	1.8 mg

SPINACH PARMESAN

(egg-free, gluten-free, sugar-free, yeast-free)   *Makes 6 servings*

Tired of plain old spinach? Here's a way to perk it up. Spinach is high in calcium, beta-carotene, and vitamin C. Dairy-free dieters may omit the cheese.

INGREDIENTS

2 pounds fresh spinach
1 garlic clove, crushed
1 tablespoon olive oil
1/8 teaspoon pepper
1/8 teaspoon nutmeg
2 tablespoons grated Parmesan cheese
6 thinly sliced red onion rings

Wash and trim spinach leaves. Mix garlic, oil, pepper, and nutmeg in a large nonstick skillet. Add washed and trimmed spinach leaves. Cover and cook over low heat until tender, adding a little more water if the water clinging to the washed leaves has completely evaporated. Mix lightly with a fork. Turn onto a serving platter and sprinkle with Parmesan cheese. Top with raw red onion rings.

NUTRITION PER SERVING

		Calories:	98		
Carbohydrate:	11 g	Cholesterol:	1.6 mg	Potassium:	518 mg
Protein:	8 g	Fiber:	2 g	Calcium:	388 mg
Total Fat:	3.8 g	Sodium:	16 mg	Iron:	1.6 mg

STEWED TOMATOES AND SPROUTS

(*dairy-free, egg-free, gluten-free, sugar-free, yeast-free*)   *Makes 6 servings*

Sprouts are so healthful. Sprinkle them on a salad or cook them as follows. This is a high vitamin C recipe.

INGREDIENTS
2 cups water
3 cups soybean sprouts
2 cups diced tomatoes
2 tablespoons chopped onion
2 tablespoons chopped green pepper
1 celery stalk, thinly sliced
1 bay leaf
¼ teaspoon dried basil
1 clove

Bring water to a boil in a large saucepan; drop sprouts in and cook 10 minutes. Remove sprouts and set aside. Pour off all but ¼ cup of the cooking liquid. Into this, add tomatoes, onion, green pepper, celery, bay leaf, basil, and clove. Cover and cook over low heat 10 minutes. Remove bay leaf and clove. Add reserved sprouts and cook 5 minutes more.

NUTRITION PER SERVING

		Calories:	37		
Carbohydrate:	8 g	Cholesterol:	0 mg	Potassium:	332 mg
Protein:	3 g	Fiber:	1 g	Calcium:	25 mg
Total Fat:	trace	Sodium:	86 mg	Iron:	1 mg

MASHED YELLOW TURNIPS

(egg-free, gluten-free, sugar-free, yeast-free)   *Makes 6 servings*

If you are bored with the same old vegetables, here's one that should pique your palate. The seasonings work without a grain of salt.

INGREDIENTS

1½ pounds yellow turnips, peeled, cut up
¼ cup skim milk
1 tablespoon corn oil margarine
1 teaspoon lemon juice
½ teaspoon grated lemon rind
¼ teaspoon nutmeg
⅛ teaspoon pepper

Cook turnips over low heat in a small amount of water in a medium size saucepan, covered, for about 20 minutes, or until soft. Drain into a medium bowl and mash. Add milk and margarine; mix well. Add lemon juice, lemon rind, nutmeg, and pepper. Mix well.

NUTRITION PER SERVING

		Calories:	38		
Carbohydrate:	4 g	Cholesterol:	.2 mg	Potassium:	164 mg
Protein:	8 g	Fiber:	.7 g	Calcium:	40 mg
Total Fat:	1.8 g	Sodium:	54 mg	Iron:	.3 mg

ZUCCHINI AND MUSHROOMS

(dairy-free, egg-free, gluten-free, sugar-free)   *Makes 4 servings*

Zucchini is rich in vitamin C. The peel is rich in fiber. Some people prefer zucchini without added tomatoes. Here's a way to combine them with mushrooms and sliced celery. It's the thyme that gives it a flavor kick! Yeast-free dieters should omit the mushrooms and add one more zucchini.

INGREDIENTS
1 teaspoon olive oil
1 small onion, finely diced
2 medium zucchini, sliced ½ inch thick
2 celery stalks, thinly sliced
¼ pound fresh mushrooms, sliced
¼ teaspoon salt
⅛ teaspoon pepper
¼ teaspoon dried thyme
¼ teaspoon paprika

Heat olive oil in a large skillet. Add onion and sauté for several minutes until golden. Add zucchini slices. Add celery, mushrooms, salt, pepper, thyme, and paprika. Stir to mix evenly. Cover and simmer over low heat for 10 minutes, or until zucchini is tender.

NUTRITION PER SERVING
Calories: 34

Carbohydrate:	6 g	Cholesterol:	0 mg	Potassium:	269 mg
Protein:	1.5 g	Fiber:	.9 g	Calcium:	39 mg
Total Fat:	1 g	Sodium:	162 mg	Iron:	.6 mg

ZUCCHINI PEPPER SKILLET

(*dairy-free, egg-free, gluten-free, sugar-free, yeast-free*)   *Makes 6 servings*

Vegetables can take on a different flavor when they are seasoned well. Here's a zucchini dish that becomes something wonderful with the addition of onion and green pepper. Try it!

INGREDIENTS
1 tablespoon olive oil
1/4 cup chopped onion
1/2 cup diced green pepper
1/4 teaspoon salt
1/8 teaspoon pepper
1/4 teaspoon dried oregano
4 cups sliced zucchini, cut 1/4 inch thick
1 tomato, cut in wedges

Heat oil in a large, nonstick skillet. Add onion, green pepper, salt, pepper, and oregano. Sauté over medium heat until vegetables are tender, about 5 minutes. Add zucchini. Cover and cook over low heat about 15 minutes, or until zucchini is tender. Stir in tomato wedges.

NUTRITION PER SERVING

		Calories:	47		
Carbohydrate:	7 g	Cholesterol:	0 mg	Potassium:	272 mg
Protein:	2 g	Fiber:	1.1 g	Calcium:	41 mg
Total Fat:	2 g	Sodium:	92 mg	Iron:	.7 mg

ZUCCHINI AND TOMATOES

(egg-free, gluten-free, sugar-free)   *Makes 4 servings*

Here's how to cook zucchini the Italian way with tomatoes and oregano as the major seasoning agents. Tuck some tiny meatballs into the pot and you'll have a whole meal!

INGREDIENTS

1 small onion, diced
1 teaspoon olive oil
1 (16-ounce) can plum tomatoes
1/4 teaspoon salt
1/8 teaspoon pepper
1/2 teaspoon dried oregano
1/4 teaspoon dried thyme
2 teaspoons grated Parmesan cheese
2 medium zucchini, sliced 1/4 inch thick

Sauté onion over medium heat in olive oil in a large, nonstick skillet, about 2 minutes. Add tomatoes, breaking up with the side of a kitchen spoon. Add salt, pepper, oregano, thyme, and cheese. Simmer covered over low heat for 10 minutes. Add sliced zucchini, cover, and simmer for 10 minutes more, or until zucchini is tender but not too soft.

NUTRITION PER SERVING

		Calories:	46		
Carbohydrate:	7 g	Cholesterol:	trace	Potassium:	296 mg
Protein:	2 g	Fiber:	.9 g	Calcium:	48 mg
Total Fat:	1 g	Sodium:	221 mg	Iron:	.7 mg

BAKED POTATO WITH CHIVE-CHEESE TOPPING

(*egg-free, gluten-free, sugar-free, yeast-free*)   *Makes 4 servings*

Instead of high-in-fat sour cream or butter, use this mixture of cottage cheese and yogurt on your potato. Just as delicious but far more nutritious!

INGREDIENTS
4 baked potatoes
½ cup 1 percent low-fat cottage cheese
1 tablespoon chopped chives
⅛ teaspoon pepper
¼ cup plain nonfat yogurt

Cut an *X* into each potato top to let the steam escape. Combine cottage cheese, chives, pepper, and yogurt in a small bowl. Beat until smooth. Serve as a topping for the potatoes.

NUTRITION PER SERVING

		Calories:	138		
Carbohydrate:	27 g	Cholesterol:	1 mg	Potassium:	650 mg
Protein:	7 g	Fiber:	.7 g	Calcium:	56 mg
Total Fat:	2 g	Sodium:	4 mg	Iron:	.9 mg

BAKED STUFFED CHEESY POTATOES

(egg-free, gluten-free, sugar-free, yeast-free)   *Makes 4 servings*

If there's anything that tastes better than a baked potato, it's a rebaked stuffed potato. Top with chopped chives if you like a mild onion flavor.

INGREDIENTS
2 baking potatoes
¼ teaspoon salt
2 tablespoons plain nonfat yogurt
1 tablespoon grated low-fat cheese
Skim milk (optional)
Paprika
Chopped chives (optional)

Bake potatoes in a 350° F oven for 1 hour. While potatoes are still hot (do use a pot holder to prevent burns) cut in half lengthwise and scoop potato out of shells without tearing the shells. Put potatoes in a medium bowl and add salt, margarine, yogurt, and cheese; whip well until potato mixture is fluffy. Add some skim milk if potatoes seem too dry. Fill reserved potato shells with the mixture, swirling the top with tines of a fork. Add a dash of paprika and a sprinkling of chives to the top of each. Potatoes may be refrigerated at this point. Just before serving, heat in a 350° F oven until tops form a lightly browned crust, about 20 minutes. Serve at once.

NUTRITION PER SERVING

		Calories:	83		
Carbohydrate:	17 g	Cholesterol:	1 mg	Potassium:	410 mg
Protein:	3 g	Fiber:	.4 g	Calcium:	43 mg
Total Fat:	.5 g	Sodium:	147 mg	Iron:	.6 mg

SCALLOPED POTATOES

(egg-free, sugar-free, yeast-free)   *Makes 4 servings*

Potatoes are a good source of potassium. Try it this way when you are already using the oven to bake another part of the meal. Let the energy do double duty!

INGREDIENTS
1 tablespoon unbleached flour
¼ teaspoon salt
⅛ teaspoon pepper
3 cups thinly sliced potatoes
1 onion, diced
1 tablespoon corn oil margarine
1 cup skim milk, scalded
¼ teaspoon paprika

Combine flour, salt, and pepper in a small bowl. Arrange a layer of potatoes in a nonstick, 1½ quart casserole. Top with some of the diced onion, then sprinkle some of the flour mixture. Dot with some of the margarine. Repeat layers, ending with a layer of potatoes. Pour scalded milk over all. Sprinkle with paprika. Cover and bake in a 350° F oven for 45 minutes; uncover and bake 15 minutes longer, or until potatoes are tender.

NUTRITION PER SERVING

		Calories:	167		
Carbohydrate:	30 g	Cholesterol:	1 mg	Potassium:	713 mg
Protein:	5 g	Fiber:	.8 g	Calcium:	92 mg
Total Fat:	2.7 g	Sodium:	205 mg	Iron:	.02 mg

BOILED DILLED POTATOES

(*dairy-free, egg-free, gluten-free, sugar-free, yeast-free*)   *Makes 2 servings*

Here's a nice trick! Boil more potatoes than you'll need for dinner, and turn the extras into potato salad for the next day. That's making one cooking stint do double time.

INGREDIENTS
6 small russet potatoes, or 2 large potatoes cut in fourths
¼ teaspoon salt
½ teaspoon dried dill
1 teaspoon corn oil margarine

Wash potatoes, but do not peel. Place potatoes in a medium saucepan; cover with water. Add salt and simmer over low heat, covered, until fork tender, about 20 minutes. Drain. Remove peels of nonrusset potatoes, but leave others on. Put potatoes into a medium bowl and toss with dill and margarine. Serve hot.

NUTRITION PER SERVING

		Calories:	106		
Carbohydrate:	20 g	Cholesterol:	0 mg	Potassium:	385 mg
Protein:	3 g	Fiber:	.7 g	Calcium:	10 mg
Total Fat:	2 g	Sodium:	292 mg	Iron:	.7 mg

ZIPPY TOMATO SALAD DRESSING

(*dairy-free, egg-free, gluten-free, sugar-free, yeast-free*)   *Makes 1 cup*

You can pep up salad greens with very few calories when you use this combination. No need to add salt—there's more than enough in regular tomato juice.

INGREDIENTS
1 cup tomato juice
2 teaspoons lemon juice
1 teaspoon grated onion
½ teaspoon prepared white horseradish
¼ teaspoon dry mustard
¼ teaspoon dried oregano

Combine all ingredients in a small bowl or jar. Serve over salad greens.

NUTRITION PER SERVING

		Calories:	3		
Carbohydrate:	.7 g	Cholesterol:	0 mg	Potassium:	36 mg
Protein:	.2 g	Fiber:	trace	Calcium:	1 mg
Total Fat:	trace	Sodium:	30 mg	Iron:	.1 mg

BUTTERMILK-DILL SALAD DRESSING

(egg-free, gluten-free, sugar-free, yeast-free)   *Makes 1 cup*

Here's a way to add extra calcium to your salad while keeping the fat content low. Try to use fresh dill if it is available.

INGREDIENTS

1 cup buttermilk
½ teaspoon celery seed
1 tablespoon fresh chopped dill, or ½ teaspoon dried
1 green onion with top, finely sliced
⅛ teaspoon salt

Combine all ingredients in a small bowl or jar and use as a dressing for salad greens.

NUTRITION PER SERVING

		Calories:	7		
Carbohydrate:	.8 g	Cholesterol:	.6 mg	Potassium:	24 mg
Protein:	.5 g	Fiber:	trace	Calcium:	18 mg
Total Fat:	.1 g	Sodium:	37 mg	Iron:	trace

ZERO SALAD DRESSING

(dairy-free, egg-free, gluten-free, sugar-free)   *Makes 1 cup*

When you are counting calories, here's the perfect dressing with no calories at all!
This is not for yeast-free dieters.

INGREDIENTS
½ cup tarragon vinegar
½ cup water
½ teaspoon dry mustard
½ teaspoon garlic powder
½ teaspoon dried oregano
¼ teaspoon white pepper

Combine all ingredients in a small bowl or jar and use as a dressing for salad greens.

NUTRITION PER SERVING
Calories: 0

Carbohydrate:	0 g	Cholesterol:	0 mg	Potassium:	7 mg
Protein:	0 g	Fiber:	0 g	Calcium:	.5 mg
Total Fat:	0 g	Sodium:	0 mg	Iron:	.05 mg

17

HEARTY GRAINS AND PASTA

$\mathbb{A}$ WHOLE GRAIN IS A GRAIN THAT HAS
not been processed, which leaves all of the nutrients intact. A processed
grain has had some of its parts removed to increase shelf life but vitamins,
minerals, and protein are removed at the same time. An enriched product
has only a few of those removed nutrients replaced. Choose a whole grain
instead of a refined grain for best benefit.

These recipes will introduce you to some grains that you may not have
used before. Cracked wheat is used in the tabbouleh recipe, kasha is also
used. Kasha is buckwheat groats and is available whole, to be cooked much
as brown rice, or ground into coarse, medium, or fine form, to be used as
flour. Kasha contains twice the amount of B vitamins as wheat and is a rich
source of potassium, phosphorus, and rutin, a substance believed to be
helpful in preventing arthritis. One-half cup of cooked kasha contains only
125 calories, packed with high-density nutrients. If you can't find it in a
supermarket, look in a health-food store or gourmet shop.

Pasta is available in over 150 shapes besides spaghetti. Select whole
wheat pasta whenever possible. Because most forms of pasta cook in about
12 minutes, it may be the best fast-food choice of all. Skip the fatty sauces
and use vegetable sauces instead.

Whole grains deliver the B vitamins needed to maintain balanced
brain chemistry. Eat your way out of depletion with whole grains!

QUICK GUIDE TO WHOLE GRAINS

- *Amaranth*. Amaranth is a seedlike grain with a peppery taste. It has
  more protein than wheat has and provides some amino acids usually
  missing in vegetable protein. Boil or steam it as a grain, eat it as a
  cereal, or pop it like popcorn.
- *Barley*. Barley has the same cholesterol-lowering benefit as oat bran,
  especially if purchased as whole-hulled barley. Whole-hulled barley
  is rich in B vitamins, protein, and fiber. Pearl barley has been

stripped of the hull and germ and, therefore, is not as nutritious as the whole grain but it is still a good source of soluble fiber.

- *Buckwheat*. Buckwheat is related to the rhubarb family and when it is roasted it has a strong nutty taste and is also known as kasha. When unroasted it is more delicately flavored and can be added to soups or cooked and served as you would brown rice.
- *Millet*. When whole hulled, millet is a tiny grain with a light beige kernel that can be cooked as a side dish or added to soups and stuffings. It is also available as puffed millet. It is rich in B vitamins.
- *Oats*. Oats are not refined in any form and, therefore, are a good source of fiber and B vitamins. It is available as rolled oats (steamed and rolled whole kernels), steel-cut oats (whole kernels that are cut into small pieces), oat groats (whole kernels), and oat bran (finely ground outer shell of the oat kernel.
- *Quinoa*. These tiny yellow seeds taste like squash when they are cooked. Quinoa is the highest in iron of all the grains; it can be cooked as a cereal, as a side dish, or added to soups. It is available in some natural-food stores.
- *Rice*. Rice is a staple food all over the world. It is best when un-polished (brown rice) with only the outer hull removed; this leaves most of the high-fiber bran layer intact. Brown rice has a nuttier flavor than polished white rice and is higher in nutrients as well. Wild rice is an unrelated grass seed and has a nutty texture that can be combined with brown rice and served as a side dish.
- *Rye*. Rye is usually ground into flour. When it is dark, it has more bran. Use rye flour to bake rye or pumpernickel bread. Whole rye berries or flakes are available in health-food stores and can be cooked as a cereal.
- *Triticale*. The whole berries or flakes of triticale can be cooked as a cereal, served as a side dish such as pilaf, or added to soups. It is a hybrid of wheat and rye, making its protein content and fiber supe-rior to wheat.
- *Wheat*. Wheat is available as whole berries, which is cooked as cereal or as a side dish or added to soups. As cracked wheat, it can be cooked into a side dish, added to ground beef, or added to soup. As bulgur (steamed, dried, and cracked into fine, medium, or coarse grinds) wheat can be served as a couscous or pilaf. When the bran is retained in bulgur, it is more nutritious. Finer grinds are used in tabbouleh. Wheat germ is the embryo of the wheat berry, rich in vitamins and minerals. Add wheat germ to meatballs, salads, or vegetables. Wheat flour is available in many different forms, as whole wheat flour, unbleached wheat flour, enriched refined flour for

fine baking, and as semolina flour for making pasta. Wheat flour has a high gluten content, however it is milled, making it an almost necessary element in baked goods.

LOW-FAT SPINACH FETTUCINE ALFREDO

(egg-free, sugar-free, yeast-free)   *Makes 4 servings*

This recipe can be made with regular fettucine but spinach fettucine gives it extra flair. Do drop a little olive oil in the cooking water to prevent the pasta from sticking.

INGREDIENTS
1 (8-ounce) package spinach fettucine
1/2 cup low-fat cottage cheese
2 tablespoons plain nonfat yogurt
2 tablespoons grated Parmesan cheese

Cook pasta according to package directions; drain well and put pasta into a large bowl. Blend cottage cheese, yogurt, and Parmesan cheese in a small bowl; toss with cooked pasta. Serve at once.

NUTRITION PER SERVING
Calories: 238

Carbohydrate:	38 g	Cholesterol:	4 mg	Potassium:	115 mg
Protein:	12 g	Fiber:	.2 g	Calcium:	89 mg
Total Fat:	3 g	Sodium:	25 mg	Iron:	1.5 mg

SALMON-PASTA SALAD

(egg-free, gluten-free, sugar-free, yeast-free)   *Makes 2 servings*

*Here's a quick meal that delivers good nutrition. Dairy-free dieters may
substitute a low-calorie salad dressing for the yogurt.*

INGREDIENTS

4 ounces small pasta shells
1½ quarts boiling water
1 (7-ounce) can salmon
1 green pepper, diced
1 carrot, grated
3 radishes, thinly sliced
¼ cup plain nonfat yogurt
1 teaspoon dried dill
¼ teaspoon dry mustard
Dash of Worcestershire sauce

Cook pasta shells in boiling water 9 to 12 minutes, until tender; drain.
Remove any skin and bones from salmon and break into chunks and drain;
put into a large bowl. Add pasta shells, green pepper, carrot, and radishes.
Combine yogurt, dill, mustard, and Worcestershire in a small bowl; mix
gently through the salmon mixture.

NUTRITION PER SERVING

		Calories:	335		
Carbohydrate:	40 g	Cholesterol:	43 mg	Potassium:	737 mg
Protein:	27 g	Fiber:	1 g	Calcium:	281 mg
Total Fat:	7 g	Sodium:	408 mg	Iron:	2.7 mg

STUFFED EGGPLANT

(egg-free, sugar-free, yeast-free)   *Makes 2 servings*

There are times when a meatless dish is most appealing. Here's one way to feel satisfied. Gluten-free dieters may substitute 1 cup of cooked rice in place of the pasta. Dairy-free dieters should omit the cheese.

INGREDIENTS
1 medium eggplant
1 small onion, diced
2 celery stalks, sliced
1/2 cup unsalted tomato juice
1/4 teaspoon dried dill
1/4 teaspoon dried oregano
1 cup cooked tiny pasta shells, drained
1 tablespoon grated Parmesan cheese

Cut eggplant in half and scoop out flesh carefully, leaving the skin unbroken; reserve skins. Dice scooped-out eggplant; place in a medium-size saucepan with onion, celery, tomato juice, dill, and oregano; simmer over low heat until tender. Remove from heat; add cooked pasta, and spoon mixture into reserved eggplant skins. Top with a sprinkling of grated cheese. Bake 20 minutes in a 350° F oven.

NUTRITION PER SERVING
Calories: 134

Carbohydrate:	25 g	Cholesterol:	2 mg	Potassium:	494 mg
Protein:	6 g	Fiber:	1.5 g	Calcium:	84 mg
Total Fat:	1.5 g	Sodium:	152 mg	Iron:	2 mg

TUNA TETRAZZINI

(egg-free, sugar-free)   *Makes 4 servings*

*Two items that should always be on the shelf are canned tuna fish and pasta.
Here they are neatly combined to produce a hot dinner for 4. Yeast-free dieters
can omit the bread crumbs.*

INGREDIENTS
2 tablespoons corn oil margarine
1 small onion, finely diced
½ green pepper, finely diced
1 tablespoon unbleached flour
1 cup skim milk
¼ teaspoon salt
⅛ teaspoon pepper
1 (7-ounce) can water-packed tuna fish, drained and flaked
8 ounces spaghetti, cooked and drained
¼ cup bread crumbs

Melt margarine in a saucepan. Sauté onion and green pepper in the margarine until onion is translucent. Stir in flour and mix until smooth and
bubbly. Gradually add milk; stirring until thick and bubbly. Add salt and
pepper. Add tuna. In a large bowl mix this sauce through the spaghetti.
Spoon into a greased, 8- × 12-inch baking dish. Top with bread crumbs.
Bake at 350° F for 25 minutes.

NUTRITION PER SERVING

		Calories:	325		
Carbohydrate:	49 g	Cholesterol:	25 mg	Potassium:	392 mg
Protein:	24 g	Fiber:	.3 g	Calcium:	111 mg
Total Fat:	7 g	Sodium:	169 mg	Iron:	2.6 mg

TUNA-NOODLE CASSEROLE

(*dairy-free, egg-free, sugar-free, yeast-free*)   *Makes 4 servings*

Here's an easy meal straight from the kitchen cupboard. It bakes while you're fixing a healthful salad.

INGREDIENTS
8 ounces broad noodles, cooked and drained
2 (7-ounce) cans water-packed tuna fish
1 (16-ounce) can unsalted tomatoes
$\frac{1}{2}$ teaspoon celery seed
$\frac{1}{4}$ teaspoon pepper
$\frac{1}{4}$ teaspoon dried thyme

Combine noodles with drained, flaked tuna in a nonstick, 1 quart casserole. Mash canned tomatoes and their liquid with celery seed, pepper, and thyme in a small bowl; pour half of this mixture over noodle mixture and toss through. Pour remaining tomato mixture over top. Bake in a 350° F oven for 25 minutes, or until top is lightly browned.

NUTRITION PER SERVING

		Calories:	344		
Carbohydrate:	41 g	Cholesterol:	154 mg	Potassium:	571 mg
Protein:	35 g	Fiber:	.7 g	Calcium:	44 mg
Total Fat:	2.5 g	Sodium:	46 mg	Iron:	3.4 mg

SPAGHETTI WITH WHITE CLAM SAUCE

(dairy-free, egg-free, sugar-free, yeast-free)   *Makes 4 servings*

You'll never be at a loss for a quick pantry meal if you keep canned minced clams and packaged spaghetti in stock. Use dried garlic and parsley, if necessary.

INGREDIENTS
1 tablespoon olive oil
2 garlic cloves, minced
1 (6½-ounce) can minced clams, including liquid
1 tablespoon chopped fresh parsley
¼ teaspoon salt
⅛ teaspoon pepper
⅛ teaspoon dried basil
8 ounces spaghetti, cooked and drained

Heat oil in a large skillet over low heat. Add garlic and brown lightly. Add clams, parsley, salt, pepper, and basil. Stir and simmer for several minutes; remove from heat. Pour over hot spaghetti in a large bowl. Toss lightly and serve at once.

NUTRITION PER SERVING

		Calories:	210		
Carbohydrate:	33 g	Cholesterol:	30 mg	Potassium:	135 mg
Protein:	9 g	Fiber:	.1 g	Calcium:	40 mg
Total Fat:	4.7 g	Sodium:	206 mg	Iron:	3 mg

SPAGHETTI WITH EGGPLANT SAUCE

(dairy-free, egg-free, sugar-free)   *Makes 2 servings*

When you are trying to keep your fat intake low, it's easy to make a vegetable sauce for pasta. Yeast-free dieters should omit the mushrooms.

INGREDIENTS
¼ pound fresh mushrooms, sliced
1 small onion, finely diced
1 small eggplant, peeled and diced
1 (8-ounce) can tomato sauce
¼ teaspoon dried oregano
¼ teaspoon dried basil
4 ounces spaghetti
1½ quarts boiling water

Place mushrooms, onion, and eggplant in a large nonstick skillet. Add tomato sauce, oregano, and basil. Cover skillet and simmer over low heat, 15 minutes, or until vegetables are soft. Meanwhile, cook spaghetti in boiling water until tender, 9 to 12 minutes. Drain and serve topped with cooked sauce.

NUTRITION PER SERVING

				Calories:	206		
Carbohydrate:	40 g	Cholesterol:	0 mg	Potassium:	597 mg
Protein:	8 g	Fiber:	1.3 g	Calcium:	40 mg
Total Fat:	1 g	Sodium:	15 mg	Iron:	2.4 mg

SPAGHETTI MILANESE

(dairy-free, egg-free, sugar-free)   *Makes 4 servings*

If you have squirreled away a few chicken livers in the freezer, now's the time to thaw them out. Use them in this piquant sauce with spaghetti. Gluten-free dieters may serve this sauce on rice. Mushrooms are a fungus so omit them for yeast-free diets.

INGREDIENTS
1 tablespoon olive oil
1 medium onion, finely diced
1/2 cup sliced fresh mushrooms
1 garlic clove, minced
8 chicken livers, cut up
1/4 teaspoon salt
1/8 teaspoon pepper
1/2 teaspoon dried oregano
1/2 teaspoon dried basil
1 (16-ounce) can tomatoes in sauce
8 ounces spaghetti, cooked and drained

Heat oil in a large, nonstick skillet. Add onion, mushrooms, and garlic; sauté over medium heat until onions are golden. Add chunks of chicken livers and brown on all sides. Add salt, pepper, oregano, and basil. Add tomatoes. Cover and simmer for 15 minutes over low heat. Serve over hot spaghetti.

NUTRITION PER SERVING
Calories: 270

Carbohydrate:	41 g	Cholesterol:	93 mg	Potassium:	501 mg
Protein:	12 g	Fiber:	.8 g	Calcium:	27 mg
Total Fat:	6.5 g	Sodium:	200 mg	Iron:	4 mg

MARINARA SAUCE

(dairy-free, egg-free, gluten-free, sugar-free, yeast-free) Makes 6 ¹/₂-cup servings.

The aroma of this simmering sauce will arouse your appetite. Use it on any kind of cooked pasta if you are not on a gluten-free diet.

INGREDIENTS
1 tablespoon olive oil
1 large onion, diced
2 garlic cloves, sliced
1 (35-ounce) can unsalted Italian tomatoes in purée
1 tablespoon chopped fresh parsley
¹/₂ teaspoon dried oregano
¹/₄ teaspoon pepper

Heat the oil in a large, nonstick skillet. Add the onions and garlic; sauté, stirring frequently, until the onion is translucent. Add tomatoes, parsley, oregano, and pepper. Reduce to low heat and simmer, covered, for 15 minutes. Press the mixture through a sieve to make a smooth sauce.

NUTRITION PER SERVING

		Calories:	52		
Carbohydrate:	10 g	Cholesterol:	0 mg	Potassium:	432 mg
Protein:	2 g	Fiber:	1 g	Calcium:	27 mg
Total Fat:	2 g	Sodium:	7 mg	Iron:	.9 mg

PASTA PRIMAVERA

(*egg-free, sugar-free, yeast-free*)   *Makes 6 servings*

Here's a dish that takes about 15 minutes to prepare. Notice that plain nonfat yogurt takes the place of cream. Those on a yeast-free diet should select frozen mixed vegetables without mushrooms.

INGREDIENTS
1 (16-ounce) package pasta spiral twists, cooked and drained
1 (16-ounce) package frozen Japanese-style vegetables (cut broccoli, green beans, onions, and green peppers), cooked
1 cup plain nonfat yogurt
2 tablespoons canned tomato paste
1/2 teaspoon salt
1/4 teaspoon pepper
1/4 teaspoon nutmeg

In a large bowl toss cooked spiral twists with cooked vegetables. Over low heat, combine yogurt, tomato paste, salt, pepper, and nutmeg, stirring until smooth and thickened; add to pasta and vegetables and toss. Serve hot.

NUTRITION PER SERVING
Calories: 232

Carbohydrate:	46 g	Cholesterol:	.6 mg	Potassium:	437 mg
Protein:	11 g	Fiber:	1.1 g	Calcium:	140 mg
Total Fat:	1 g	Sodium:	8 mg	Iron:	2 mg

CHICKEN AND MACARONI SALAD

(egg-free, sugar-free, yeast-free)   *Makes 2 servings*

If you have a cup of left-over cooked chicken, here's a delicious way to stretch it into a satisfying meal. Dairy-free dieters may substitute a light salad dressing for the yogurt.

INGREDIENTS
4 ounces macaroni
1½ quarts boiling water
1 cup cubed cooked chicken
¼ cup frozen peas, thawed
1 carrot, finely diced
2 celery stalks, finely diced
1 tablespoon finely diced onion
½ cup plain nonfat yogurt
1 teaspoon grated lemon peel
½ teaspoon dried dill

Cook macaroni in boiling water 9 to 12 minutes until tender; drain. Combine macaroni with chicken, peas, carrot, celery, and onion in a large bowl. Stir together yogurt, lemon peel, and dill in a small bowl and mix through the chicken mixture.

NUTRITION PER SERVING

		Calories:	324		
Carbohydrate:	40 g	Cholesterol:	31 mg	Potassium:	697 mg
Protein:	26 g	Fiber:	1 g	Calcium:	165 mg
Total Fat:	3 g	Sodium:	119 mg	Iron:	2.9 mg

NOODLE PUDDING

(sugar-free)   *Makes 8 servings*

This is called a pudding but it's a solid pasta and protein offering. You can use it as a main course for lunch, a side dish for dinner, or as a buffet offering. Make plenty—it'll go like hotcakes! Yeast-free dieters should omit bread crumbs.

INGREDIENTS
1 (8-ounce) package medium width noodles
2 eggs
1 cup low-fat cottage cheese
1 cup plain nonfat yogurt
1/4 teaspoon salt
2 tablespoons lemon juice
1/2 cup seedless white raisins
2 tablespoons corn oil margarine
1/4 cup fine unseasoned bread crumbs

Cook noodles according to package directions; drain. Beat eggs in a large bowl; add cottage cheese and sour cream and beat well. Add salt, lemon juice, and raisins. Fold cooked, drained noodles into this mixture. Spoon into an 8 × 12-inch nonstick baking pan. Dot top with margarine and sprinkle with bread crumbs. Bake for 45 minutes at 350° F. Serve hot or cold.

NUTRITION PER SERVING
Calories: 240

Carbohydrate:	32 g	Cholesterol:	71 mg	Potassium:	252 mg
Protein:	16 g	Fiber:	.2 g	Calcium:	117 mg
Total Fat:	6 g	Sodium:	143 mg	Iron:	1.5 mg

LASAGNE

(sugar-free, yeast-free)   *Makes 8 main-course servings*

Although this may take some extra time to prepare, it is an excellent choice to make for a casual supper for guests. It also takes kindly to freezing and reheating, which may be a good reason to make a panful for yourself and then coast on the goodness of it for several months to come.

INGREDIENTS
1 pound lean ground beef
1 large onion, finely diced

2 garlic cloves, finely diced
1 teaspoon dried basil
1 teaspoon dried oregano
$1/2$ teaspoon salt
$1/4$ teaspoon pepper
1 (30-ounce) can tomatoes in sauce
1 (6-ounce) can tomato paste
1 (8-ounce) package lasagne noodles, cooked and drained
2 cups low-fat ricotta cheese
1 egg
$1/2$ pound low-fat mozzarella cheese, sliced thin
$1/2$ cup grated Parmesan cheese

Break beef into bits and brown over medium heat in a large nonstick skillet; break apart further with a fork as it browns. Add onion, garlic, basil, oregano, salt, and pepper. Add tomatoes and tomato paste; stir well. Cover and simmer for 20 minutes. Spoon a thin layer of sauce over the bottom of a 8 × 11-inch nonstick baking dish. Top with a side-by-side layer of lasagne noodles; use one-third of the noodles. Combine ricotta cheese and egg in a small bowl. Spread one-half of the ricotta mixture over the noodles. Top with one-third of the mozzarella cheese and sprinkle with one-third of the Parmesan cheese. Top with a layer of one-half of the remaining noodles. Top with remaining ricotta mixture and one-half of the remaining mozzarella slices, then sprinkle with one-half of the remaining Parmesan. Top with the remaining noodles. Spread remaining meat sauce over all. Place remaining mozzarella slices evenly over the top and sprinkle with remaining Parmesan. Bake in a 350° F oven for 45 minutes.

NUTRITION PER SERVING

		Calories:	376		
Carbohydrate:	28 g	Cholesterol:	107 mg	Potassium:	628 mg
Protein:	29 g	Fiber:	.7 g	Calcium:	363 mg
Total Fat:	16 g	Sodium:	409 mg	Iron:	3.4 mg

MEATLESS LASAGNE

(*sugar-free, yeast-free*)   *Makes 8 servings*

The main ingredients in this dish are a package of lasagne noodles and a pint of ricotta cheese. The rest should be available in your refrigerator and pantry shelf. Whip this up when you're expecting 4 or more people and don't want to go out marketing to serve them.

INGREDIENTS
1 (16-ounce) package lasagne noodles
1 tablespoon finely diced onion
1 green pepper, seeded and finely diced
1 (29-ounce) can tomatoes in sauce, cut up
1/2 teaspoon dried oregano
1/4 teaspoon garlic powder
2 cups low-fat ricotta cheese
1 egg
1/2 cup grated Parmesan cheese

Cook lasagne noodles according to package directions, drain. Heat oil in a large, nonstick skillet. Sauté onion and green pepper over medium heat for several minutes. Add tomatoes, oregano, and garlic powder. Reduce heat, cover and simmer for 10 minutes. Spread a thin layer of sauce over the bottom of a 9 × 12-inch baking dish. Arrange a layer of one-third of the lasagne noodles side-by-side over the sauce. Combine ricotta cheese and egg in a small bowl, beating well. Spread a layer of one-half of the ricotta mixture over the noodles. Sprinkle with one-third of the Parmesan cheese. Arrange one-half of the remaining noodles over this; top with remaining ricotta mixture and sprinkle with one-half of the remaining Parmesan. Arrange remaining noodles over top; spoon remaining sauce over all. Sprinkle with remaining Parmesan. Bake in a 350° F oven for 30 minutes.

NUTRITION PER SERVING
Calories: 221

Carbohydrate:	24 g	Cholesterol:	58 mg	Potassium:	352 mg
Protein:	14 g	Fiber:	.5 g	Calcium:	268 mg
Total Fat:	8 g	Sodium:	173 mg	Iron:	1.6 mg

COTTAGE CHEESE LASAGNE

(*egg-free, sugar-free, yeast-free*)   *Makes 8 servings*

This is the way to keep the fat calories low while enjoying a cheese-filled pasta dish. Read the labels carefully when purchasing low-fat dairy products. Look for the lowest possible fat content.

INGREDIENTS

8 ounces lasagne noodles
2 cups tomato sauce
$1/4$ teaspoon garlic powder
$1/2$ teaspoon dried oregano
$1/8$ teaspoon pepper
2 cups 1 percent low-fat cottage cheese
$1/2$ cup shredded low-fat mozzarella cheese
1 cup plain nonfat yogurt
$1/4$ cup sliced scallions, green part included
$1/2$ cup chopped green pepper
2 tablespoons grated Parmesan cheese

Cook noodles according to package directions; drain. Combine tomato sauce, garlic powder, oregano, and pepper in a medium bowl. Combine cottage cheese, mozzarella cheese, yogurt, scallions, and green pepper in another medium bowl; mix well. Spread half of the cooked lasagne noodles side-by-side in a 13 × 9 × 2-inch nonstick baking dish. Cover with a thin layer of tomato mixture. Cover with the cottage cheese mixture. Top with remaining noodles, then cover all with remaining tomato mixture. Sprinkle with Parmesan cheese. Bake in a 375° F oven for 40 minutes. Allow to stand 10 minutes before serving.

NUTRITION PER SERVING

		Calories:	195		
Carbohydrate:	28 g	Cholesterol:	9 mg	Potassium:	361 mg
Protein:	15 g	Fiber:	.5 g	Calcium:	171 mg
Total Fat:	2.7 g	Sodium:	15 mg	Iron:	1.2 mg

STUFFED BAKED MANICOTTI

(egg-free, sugar-free)   *Makes 6 servings*

All meals need not include meat as long as there is some source of protein available. In this recipe, the protein is in the cheese. This takes a little fussing, but it's worth it! Yeast-free dieters should omit the bread crumb topping.

INGREDIENTS
1 (16-ounce) package manicotti
1 pound low-fat ricotta cheese
3 tablespoons grated Parmesan cheese
$\frac{1}{2}$ teaspoon salt
1 tablespoon chopped dill
1 (16-ounce) can tomatoes in sauce
2 tablespoons tomato paste
$\frac{1}{2}$ cup Italian-seasoned bread crumbs

Cook manicotti according to package directions; remove from water as soon as pasta is pliable. Combine ricotta cheese, Parmesan cheese, salt, and dill in a medium bowl. Blend tomatoes and tomato paste in a blender. Stuff cooked noodle tubes with cheese mixture and place side-by-side in a greased, flat, 8 × 12-inch baking dish. Spoon tomato sauce over stuffed manicotti. Top with bread crumbs. Bake in a 350° F oven for 30 minutes, or until pasta is very tender.

NUTRITION PER SERVING
Calories: 340

Carbohydrate:	47 g	Cholesterol:	27 mg	Potassium:	465 mg
Protein:	18 g	Fiber:	.6 g	Calcium:	294 mg
Total Fat:	8 g	Sodium:	418 mg	Iron:	2.6 mg

RICE AND CARROT RING

(gluten-free, sugar-free, yeast-free)   *Makes 6 servings*

This method of cooking the rice in a pan of water is the best way to keep it moist. To serve, turn ring pan upside down and tap gently, much like making mud pies!

INGREDIENTS
2 cups cooked brown rice
1 cup grated carrots
1/4 cup grated Parmesan cheese
2 eggs, beaten
1/2 teaspoon salt
1/4 teaspoon pepper
1/4 teaspoon dried dill

Combine rice, carrots, and cheese in a large bowl. Stir in eggs, salt, pepper, and dill. Spoon into a nonstick 1-quart ring mold. Place in a pan of hot water and bake in a 350° F oven for 25 minutes.

NUTRITION PER SERVING

		Calories:	128		
Carbohydrate:	18 g	Cholesterol:	95 mg	Potassium:	134 mg
Protein:	8 g	Fiber:	.9 g	Calcium:	82 mg
Total Fat:	3 g	Sodium:	420 mg	Iron:	.8 mg

RICE AND MUSHROOM RING

(dairy-free, egg-free, gluten-free, sugar-free)   *Makes 6 servings*

Brown rice is preferable to white because it is a whole grain. The rice may be cooked and packed into the mold earlier in the day, then set into a pan of hot water and heated in the oven for 20 minutes, or until warmed through. Yeast-free dieters can omit the mushrooms.

INGREDIENTS
2 teaspoons olive oil
½ pound fresh mushrooms, sliced
1 onion, diced
1 green pepper, diced
1 (16-ounce) can tomatoes
½ cup (or more) water
1 cup uncooked brown rice
2 tablespoons chopped parsley
½ teaspoon salt

Heat oil in a large deep saucepan. Add mushrooms, onion, and green pepper and sauté over medium heat until limp. Drain tomatoes, reserving the liquid; add tomatoes to saucepan. Measure reserved liquid and add water to make a total of 2 cups. Add liquid to saucepan, stir, and bring to a boil. Add rice, parsley, and salt. Turn heat to low, cover, and cook for 30 minutes, stirring once during the cooking time. Pack into a nonstick 1-quart ring mold and turn out onto a platter. Serve hot.

NUTRITION PER SERVING
Calories: 152

Carbohydrate:	30 g	Cholesterol:	0 mg	Potassium:	345 mg
Protein:	4 g	Fiber:	1.4 g	Calcium:	24 mg
Total Fat:	2 g	Sodium:	290 mg	Iron:	1.2 mg

RICE AMANDINE

(dairy-free, egg-free, gluten-free, sugar-free, yeast-free)   *Makes 6 servings*

Almonds give this dish a bit of crunch. Fancy enough for company dinner!

INGREDIENTS
1 cup uncooked brown rice
6 scallions with tops, thinly sliced

2½ cups fat-free chicken broth
2 tablespoons chopped fresh parsley
¼ cup slivered almonds

Combine rice, scallions, broth, and parsley in a large, heavy saucepan. Bring to a boil; stir once, then reduce heat to low. Cover and simmer for 20 minutes, or until liquid is absorbed. Remove from heat, add almonds and fluff lightly with a fork.

NUTRITION PER SERVING

		Calories:	146		
Carbohydrate:	25 g	Cholesterol:	0 mg	Potassium:	128 mg
Protein:	3 g	Fiber:	1.2 g	Calcium:	20 mg
Total Fat:	3 g	Sodium:	4 mg	Iron:	.8 mg

GREEN RICE

(dairy-free, egg-free, gluten-free, sugar-free, yeast-free)   *Makes 6 servings*

All the greenery perks up the rice. Brown rice gives you essential B-complex vitamins. Good for brain power!

INGREDIENTS
1 cup uncooked brown rice
6 scallions with tops, thinly sliced
1 green pepper, seeded and finely diced
3 tablespoons chopped fresh parsley
2 cups fat-free chicken broth
¼ teaspoon white pepper

Combine all ingredients in a 2-quart casserole. Cover with a tight-fitting lid or foil. Bake 30 minutes in a 350° F oven, or until rice is tender and liquid is absorbed. Toss lightly with a fork before serving.

NUTRITION PER SERVING

		Calories:	116		
Carbohydrate:	25 g	Cholesterol:	0 mg	Potassium:	116 mg
Protein:	2 g	Fiber:	1.2 g	Calcium:	12 mg
Total Fat:	.5 g	Sodium:	6 mg	Iron:	.5 mg

HOT CRABMEAT ON RICE

(dairy-free, egg-free, gluten-free, sugar-free)   *Makes 2 servings*

If you keep a can of crabmeat on your staple shelf, you will always have the makings of a quick meal. If there's no time to cook rice, packaged croutons or toast points can be a good base for those who are not gluten-free or yeast-free dieters.

INGREDIENTS
1 tablespoon olive oil
1 small onion, diced fine
1 tablespoon chopped fresh parsley
2 garlic cloves, diced fine
1 (7-ounce) can crabmeat, cut up
1 cup cooked enriched white rice

Heat oil in a nonstick skillet. Add onion, parsley, and garlic; sauté for several minutes, until onion is limp. Then add crabmeat chunks, and cook to heat through, gently turning with a spoon to coat with the onion mixture. Serve at once over cooked rice.

NUTRITION PER SERVING

		Calories:	250		
Carbohydrate:	28 g	Cholesterol:	69 mg	Potassium:	115 mg
Protein:	14 g	Fiber:	.3 g	Calcium:	51 mg
Total Fat:	8 g	Sodium:	333 mg	Iron:	1.6 mg

LENTIL-RICE CASSEROLE

(dairy-free, egg-free, sugar-free)   *Makes 6 servings*

Not all protein is derived from meat, fish, poultry, eggs, and cheese. When you mix a legume together with a grain, you combine their amino acids into the essential group that your body needs every day for growth and repair. Gluten-free and yeast-free dieters may omit the bread crumbs.

INGREDIENTS
$^2/_3$ cup lentils
1 cup uncooked brown rice
3 cups water
2 tablespoons olive oil
1 medium onion, diced
1 garlic clove, minced
5 celery stalks, finely diced
$2^1/_2$ cups canned tomatoes
$^1/_2$ teaspoon salt
$^1/_4$ teaspoon pepper
1 teaspoon dried dill
$^1/_2$ cup whole wheat bread crumbs

Soak lentils in water to cover overnight. Simmer lentils slowly in the soaking water until tender, about 2 hours. Drain, reserving liquid. Place rice and the 3 cups water in a medium saucepan; bring to a boil, then reduce heat, cover, and simmer for 20 minutes, fluffing once with a fork during the cooking time. In the meantime, heat oil in a large saucepan and add onion, garlic, and celery; sauté over medium heat until vegetables are soft, about 7 minutes. Add tomatoes and lentils with $^1/_2$ cup of the reserved cooking water. Add cooked rice, salt, pepper, and dill. Mix well. Sprinkle a thin coating of bread crumbs over a greased 2-quart baking dish, and fill with lentil–rice mixture. Top with remaining bread crumbs. Bake for 30 minutes in a 350° F oven.

NUTRITION PER SERVING

		Calories:	256		
Carbohydrate:	43 g	Cholesterol:	0 mg	Potassium:	533 mg
Protein:	76 g	Fiber:	2 g	Calcium:	47 mg
Total Fat:	75 g	Sodium:	414 mg	Iron:	2.3 mg

KASHA PILAF WITH MUSHROOMS

(dairy-free, gluten-free, sugar-free)   *Makes 6 servings*

Kasha is buckwheat groats and does not contain gluten. It has an interesting nutty flavor, although it is a grain. Serve it in place of rice or potatoes. Yeast-free dieters should omit the mushrooms.

INGREDIENTS

1 cup uncooked whole or coarse kasha
1 egg white, lightly beaten
$1/4$ teaspoon nutmeg
1 tablespoon olive oil
1 cup thinly sliced celery
$1/2$ cup chopped onion
2 cups hot fat-free chicken broth
$1/4$ pound fresh mushrooms, sliced
2 tablespoons chopped fresh parsley

In a large nonstick skillet, combine kasha, egg white, and nutmeg. Stir constantly over low heat until each grain is separate and dry. Push kasha to one side. Add oil, celery, and onion; sauté briefly, then stir into kasha. Add hot broth, cover pan tightly and simmer over low heat for 15 minutes, or until kasha grains are tender and most of the liquid is absorbed. In a separate small skillet, sauté mushrooms and parsley over medium heat in a few tablespoons of water, until mushrooms are limp; add to kasha and stir well.

NUTRITION PER SERVING

		Calories:	142		
Carbohydrate:	26 g	Cholesterol:	0 mg	Potassium:	184 mg
Protein:	3 g	Fiber:	1 g	Calcium:	25 mg
Total Fat:	2.7 g	Sodium:	39 mg	Iron:	.7 mg

TUNA-KASHA SALAD

(gluten-free, sugar-free, yeast-free)   *Makes 3 servings*

Here's another healthy way to stretch a can of tuna fish into a hearty salad. Kasha is a buckwheat product, contains no gluten, and is actually related to rhubarb! When cooked according to package directions, it forms a bulky crunchy grain with a nutlike flavor.

INGREDIENTS
1 (7-ounce) can water-packed tuna fish, drained
3/4 cup cooked kasha
2 hard-cooked eggs, chopped
1/4 cup chopped celery
1/4 cup chopped onion
2 tablespoons chopped green pepper
1/4 cup plain nonfat yogurt
1 tablespoon prepared mustard
2 teaspoons lemon juice

Combine tuna and kasha in a medium bowl. Add eggs, celery, onion, and green pepper. Mix together yogurt, mustard, and lemon juice in a small bowl. Toss with tuna mixture. Chill.

NUTRITION PER SERVING
Calories: 214

Carbohydrate:	16 g	Cholesterol:	183 mg	Potassium:	384 mg
Protein:	25 g	Fiber:	.6 g	Calcium:	82 mg
Total Fat:	4 g	Sodium:	220 mg	Iron:	2.2 mg

TABBOULEH

(dairy-free, egg-free, sugar-free, yeast-free)   *Makes 6 servings*

Bulgur is parboiled cracked wheat. It is usually soaked and either eaten raw in a salad or cooked in liquid as a side dish. Either way, it is very nutritious. Here it is as a cold salad.

INGREDIENTS
1 cup bulgur
2 tomatoes, finely diced
1 sweet Italian pepper, finely diced
1 cucumber, seeded and finely diced
2 green onions, including tops, finely sliced
2 tablespoons chopped fresh parsley
2 teaspoons chopped fresh mint leaves
1/4 cup olive oil
1/4 cup lemon juice
1/4 teaspoon pepper

Place bulgur in a medium bowl and cover with water. Let stand for at least 1 hour. Drain bulgur, squeeze dry, and return to bowl. Add tomatoes, Italian pepper, cucumber, scallions, parsley, and mint. Fluff all together with a fork. Combine olive oil, lemon juice, and pepper; pour over bulgur mixture and mix through. Chill until ready to serve.

NUTRITION PER SERVING

		Calories:	200		
Carbohydrate:	27 g	Cholesterol:	0 mg	Potassium:	244 mg
Protein:	3 g	Fiber:	.8 g	Calcium:	21 mg
Total Fat:	9 g	Sodium:	5 mg	Iron:	1.8 mg

BULGUR PILAF

(dairy-free, egg-free, sugar-free, yeast-free)   *Makes 8 servings*

Here is the bulgur (cracked wheat) baked in broth to produce a delicious pilaf. This same method can be used to bake a simple brown rice pilaf, for those who are on a gluten-free diet.

INGREDIENTS
1 medium onion, finely diced
1 tablespoon olive oil
2 cups bulgur
4 cups fat-free chicken broth
1 tablespoon fresh chopped parsley
1/4 teaspoon pepper

Using a small, nonstick skillet, sauté diced onion in olive oil over medium heat, stirring constantly, until onion is translucent. Combine bulgur and chicken broth in a large baking pan with a tight cover. Add the sautéed onion, the parsley, and pepper. Stir well. Bake 30 minutes at 350° F, tightly covered, then fluff with a fork and bake an additional 15 minutes.

NUTRITION PER SERVING

		Calories:	176		
Carbohydrate:	36 g	Cholesterol:	0 mg	Potassium:	135 mg
Protein:	4 g	Fiber:	.6 g	Calcium:	17 mg
Total Fat:	2 g	Sodium:	1 mg	Iron:	2.1 mg

COUSCOUS

(dairy-free, egg-free, sugar-free, yeast-free)   *Makes 4 servings*

This cracked wheat dish can be served hot or cold. Mint leaves give an unusual flavor. Gluten-free dieters may use brown rice as a substitute for the cracked wheat.

INGREDIENTS

1 tablespoon olive oil
1 large onion, finely diced
1/2 cup grated carrots
1/2 cup fat-free chicken broth
2 cups cooked couscous (cracked durum wheat)
1/4 cup seedless white raisins
1 tablespoon lemon juice
1/8 teaspoon pepper
1 tablespoon chopped fresh mint leaves

Heat olive oil in a large, nonstick skillet and sauté onion over medium heat until it is translucent. Add carrots and chicken broth. Lower temperature, cover and cook 5 minutes. Place couscous in a deep bowl. Add raisins, lemon juice, pepper, and mint. Pour broth mixture into couscous and toss lightly with a fork. Serve hot or refrigerate until ready to serve.

NUTRITION PER SERVING

		Calories:	186		
Carbohydrate:	35 g	Cholesterol:	0 mg	Potassium:	221 mg
Protein:	3 g	Fiber:	1 g	Calcium:	28 mg
Total Fat:	3 g	Sodium:	286 mg	Iron:	1 mg

18

MUFFINS AND QUICK BREADS

$\mathbb{M}$IXED MESSAGES ABOUND IN HEALTH
communications. Choosing a bran muffin often results in choosing a load of
fat and sugar with the bran. Whole-grain breads may not deliver the
nutrients you desire—read labels to be sure you are getting a nutritious
mouthful. Better yet, bake your own.

There's something for everyone in this chapter. Yeast-free dieters will
be able to bake batter breads. Gluten-free dieters who yearn for a slice of
bread will be able to bake with nongluten flour and to adapt some of their
own recipes using the grain equivalency chart. Don't expect to find the
resiliency or the keepability of a gluten flour product in a nongluten
product. Sometimes it requires a combination of several nongluten flours to
produce a satisfactory texture. Adding a banana often does the trick.

It's easy to stir up quick batter breads and muffins. Use nonstick pans
and paper muffin liners to reduce the need for greasing the pans. Always
preheat the oven before you start to mix the batter, to get a more evenly
baked product.

Some brown sugar, molasses, or honey appears in these breads and
muffins. Keep in mind that there are sixteen tablespoons to a cup, and
three teaspoons to a tablespoon. When these natural sweeteners are divided among the serving portions, each serving has a minimal amount.
Also, when one or two eggs are divided among a dozen servings, the
amount of yolk is minimal in each. All other fat used is vegetable-based and
limited as much as possible. Whichever recipe you choose, you will be
baking with less fat, no white sugar, and reduced sodium!

GRAIN EQUIVALENCY TABLE

Substitutions for 1 cup wheat flour for baking*
  1 cup corn flour
  3/4 cup coarse cornmeal
  3/4 cup plus 3 tablespoons fine cornmeal
  1/2 cup plus 2 tablespoons potato starch flour

247

¾ cup plus 2 tablespoons rice flour
1 cup soybean flour plus ¼ cup potato starch flour
1 cup millet meal
Substitutions for 1 tablespoon wheat flour for thickening
  ½ tablespoon cornstarch
  ½ tablespoon potato starch flour
  ½ tablespoon rice flour
  ½ tablespoon arrowroot starch
  2 teaspoons quick-cooking tapioca
  1 tablespoon millet meal

* Add 1 egg to recipe if it contains less than 2 cups wheat flour.

Source: The Allergic Gourmet, June Roth, M.S. (1983), Contemporary Books.

APPLESAUCE MUFFINS

(yeast-free)   *Makes 1 dozen muffins*

Remember to use paper-lined muffin tins so you can skip the chore of greasing the muffin pan. This recipe can be thrown together in a few minutes; then you can enjoy the whiffs of fresh baking for 30 minutes before enjoying the goodies.

INGREDIENTS
2 cups unbleached flour
3 tablespoons brown sugar
1 tablespoon baking powder
½ teaspoon salt
1 egg
1 cup skim milk
¼ cup corn oil
1 cup unsweetened applesauce

Combine flour, sugar, baking powder, and salt in a large bowl; stir to mix well. In a small bowl, beat egg lightly. Add milk and corn oil to the egg; beat until well mixed. Make a well in the middle of the flour mixture and pour milk mixture into it. Add applesauce. Stir lightly, until flour is well moistened. Batter will be lumpy. Spoon into muffin tins, filling cups two-thirds full. Bake in a preheated 350° F oven for 30 minutes, or until lightly browned.

NUTRITION PER MUFFIN

		Calories:	151		
Carbohydrate:	22 g	Cholesterol:	23 mg	Potassium:	87 mg
Protein:	4 g	Fiber:	.2 g	Calcium:	49 mg
Total Fat:	5 g	Sodium:	188 mg	Iron:	.1 mg

BRAN MUFFINS

(yeast-free) *Makes 1 dozen muffins*

It's wise to increase the amount of bran in the diet to give extra fiber and extra flavor. This recipe is health conscious in other ways—note the skim milk and small amount of shortening.

INGREDIENTS

1½ cups unbleached flour
1 tablespoon baking powder
1 teaspoon salt
½ cup brown sugar
1½ cups all-bran cereal
1 cup skim milk
1 egg
⅓ cup vegetable shortening

Sift together the flour, baking powder, salt, and sugar into a medium bowl. In a large bowl stir together the all-bran cereal and milk; let stand for several minutes until most of the liquid is absorbed by the cereal. Then add egg and shortening and beat well. Stir in the flour mixture only until well combined. Fill paper-lined muffin cups three-quarters full. Bake in a preheated 400° F oven for 25 minutes, or until muffins are golden brown.

NUTRITION PER MUFFIN

		Calories:	148		
Carbohydrate:	21 g	Cholesterol:	23 mg	Potassium:	53 mg
Protein:	2 g	Fiber:	.05 g	Calcium:	28 mg
Total Fat:	6 g	Sodium:	268 mg	Iron:	.6 mg

OATMEAL MUFFINS

(yeast-free)   *Makes 1 dozen muffins*

This is a nutritious muffin for those who are not sensitive to its ingredients. If you use fluted paper liners in the muffin tins you won't have to grease them. Clean-up goes easier, too!

INGREDIENTS
1 cup unbleached flour
2 teaspoons baking powder
1/2 teaspoon baking soda
1/2 teaspoon salt
1/4 teaspoon cinnamon
1 cup uncooked oatmeal
1/2 cup brown sugar
1 cup buttermilk
1 egg
1/4 cup salad oil

Sift together unbleached flour, baking powder, baking soda, salt, and cinnamon into a medium bowl. Combine oatmeal and brown sugar in a large bowl. Add buttermilk and stir well. Beat together egg and salad oil; add to oatmeal mixture. Add sifted ingredients and mix just until all ingredients are moistened. Spoon mixture into paper-lined muffin cups, filling cups two-thirds full. Bake in a preheated 375° F oven for 25 minutes, or until lightly browned.

NUTRITION PER MUFFIN
Calories: 138

Carbohydrate:	20 g	Cholesterol:	23 mg	Potassium:	91 mg
Protein:	3 g	Fiber:	.07 g	Calcium:	47 mg
Total Fat:	5 g	Sodium:	222 mg	Iron:	.8 mg

WHOLE WHEAT YOGURT MUFFINS

(*yeast-free*)   *Makes 1 dozen muffins*

This is an excellent muffin that is chock-full of healthy ingredients. Spoon into paper-lined muffin cups and skip the necessity to grease the pan.

INGREDIENTS

1 cup whole wheat graham flour
3/4 cup wheat germ
3 tablespoons brown sugar
1/2 teaspoon baking powder
1/2 teaspoon baking soda
1/2 teaspoon salt
1 egg, lightly beaten
1 cup plain nonfat yogurt
6 tablespoons melted corn oil margarine

In a large bowl combine flour, wheat germ, sugar, baking powder, baking soda, and salt. Combine egg, yogurt, and melted margarine in a medium bowl and mix well. Pour into flour mixture and stir just enough to blend all ingredients. Mixture may be lumpy. Pour into paper-lined muffin cups. Fill two-thirds full. Bake in a preheated 375° F oven for 20 to 25 minutes, or until a wooden toothpick inserted into the center comes out clean.

NUTRITION PER MUFFIN

		Calories:	137		
Carbohydrate:	15 g	Cholesterol:	23 mg	Potassium:	161 mg
Protein:	5 g	Fiber:	1 g	Calcium:	54 mg
Total Fat:	7 g	Sodium:	88 mg	Iron:	1 mg

BUTTERMILK BISCUITS

(egg-free, sugar-free, yeast-free)   *Makes 1 dozen biscuits*

If you place the biscuits on the baking sheet so that they touch each other, they will come out soft. If you prefer them crispy, place them farther apart. Be gentle when kneading the dough, this will produce a tender biscuit.

INGREDIENTS
2 cups sifted unbleached flour
1 tablespoon baking powder
1/2 teaspoon salt
1/2 teaspoon baking soda
1/3 cup corn oil
1/3 cup buttermilk

Stir together flour, baking powder, salt, and baking soda in a large bowl. Blend in oil with a fork. Stir in buttermilk. Mix until dough forms into a ball. Knead dough on a lightly floured board for 1 minute. Roll or pat out to a 1/2-inch thickness. Cut with a floured biscuit cutter or the floured rim of a glass. Place on an ungreased cookie sheet. Bake in a preheated 450° F oven for 12 to 15 minutes, or until lightly browned.

NUTRITION PER BISCUIT
Calories: 127

Carbohydrate:	15 g	Cholesterol:	.2 mg	Potassium:	30 mg
Protein:	2 g	Fiber:	.05 g	Calcium:	26 mg
Total Fat:	6 g	Sodium:	180 mg	Iron:	.5 mg

BANANA BRAN BREAD

(dairy-free, yeast-free)   *Makes 1 loaf; 16 slices*

Whole grains add bulk to the diet, an important factor in preventing colon disorders. This is a good recipe to remember when you have some very ripe bananas. This banana bread is not for hypoglycemics because of its sugar content.

INGREDIENTS
1 cup unbleached flour
½ cup whole wheat flour
½ cup bran cereal
1 teaspoon baking powder
½ teaspoon baking soda
½ teaspoon salt
½ cup shortening
¼ cup light brown sugar
1 cup mashed bananas
1 egg

Sift the flours, bran, baking powder, baking soda, and salt in a medium bowl. In a large bowl beat shortening and sugar together until fluffy. Add banana and egg; beat well. Gradually add sifted dry ingredients to banana mixture. Beat well. Pour batter into a 9×5-inch nonstick loaf pan. Bake in a preheated 350° F oven for 50 to 60 minutes. Bread is done when toothpick inserted in the center comes out dry. Remove from the oven and cool in the pan for 10 minutes. Remove from pan and finish cooling.

NUTRITION PER SLICE

		Calories:	123		
Carbohydrate:	14 g	Cholesterol:	17 mg	Potassium:	105 mg
Protein:	2 g	Fiber:	.5 g	Calcium:	9 mg
Total Fat:	7 g	Sodium:	102 mg	Iron:	.7 mg

MOLASSES BROWN BREAD

(*dairy-free*)   *Makes 1 loaf; 16 slices*

This is a nutritious loaf of bread with a spicy flavor. Reminiscent of New England hearty loaves, it all goes together in a matter of minutes! Yeast-free and sugar-free dieters should omit this recipe because of the molasses.

INGREDIENTS
1 cup unbleached flour
1 teaspoon baking powder
1/2 teaspoon baking soda
1/2 teaspoon salt
1/2 teaspoon cinnamon
1 cup all-bran cereal
1/2 cup seedless raisins
2 tablespoons vegetable shortening
1/3 cup molasses
3/4 cup boiling water
1 egg

Sift together flour, baking powder, baking soda, salt, and cinnamon into a medium bowl. Combine bran cereal, raisins, shortening, and molasses in a large bowl. Add boiling water, stirring until shortening is melted. Add egg and beat well. Gradually add sifted ingredients and stir only until all the ingredients are moistened. Pour batter into a nonstick 9×5-inch loaf pan. Bake in preheated 350° F oven for 35 to 45 minutes, or until browned. Test with a toothpick for doneness.

NUTRITION PER SLICE

		Calories:	85		
Carbohydrate:	16 g	Cholesterol:	17 mg	Potassium:	123 mg
Protein:	2 g	Fiber:	.1 g	Calcium:	23 mg
Total Fat:	2 g	Sodium:	114 mg	Iron:	1.1 mg

WHEAT-FREE BANANA BREAD

(dairy-free, gluten-free, yeast-free)   *Makes 1 loaf; 12 slices*

Batter breads are easy to make. This one should be welcome to those who are gluten-free dieters. The mix of rice flour and potato flour, combined with banana gives it a reasonable texture. Potato flour is sometimes labeled potato starch.

INGREDIENTS
1½ cups rice flour
1 cup potato flour
1 tablespoon baking powder
1⅓ cups mashed banana
½ cup light brown sugar
½ teaspoon salt
2 eggs, beaten
½ cup corn oil
2 tablespoons water

Sift together flours and baking powder into a medium bowl. In a large bowl, combine banana, sugar, and salt; add eggs, oil, and water. Mix well. Stir in dry ingredients and mix well. Spoon into a nonstick 8×4-inch loaf pan. Let stand at room temperature for 5 minutes before placing in a preheated 350° F oven. Bake for 1 hour. Transfer loaf from pan onto a rack to cool.

NUTRITION PER SLICE

		Calories:	210		
Carbohydrate:	26 g	Cholesterol:	46 mg	Potassium:	99 mg
Protein:	4 g	Fiber:	.1 g	Calcium:	25 mg
Total Fat:	11 g	Sodium:	135 mg	Iron:	1 mg

CORN BREAD

(gluten-free, yeast-free)   *Makes 12 servings*

If you are on a gluten-free diet, here's a corn bread recipe that is made without the usual wheat flour. If you buy corn bread or any cornmeal products, read the label carefully—wheat is usually included.

INGREDIENTS
2 cups cornmeal
1 tablespoon baking powder
$1/2$ teaspoon salt
1 egg
1 cup skim milk
$1/4$ cup corn oil
1 tablespoon honey

Combine cornmeal, baking powder, and salt in a medium bowl. Beat egg in a large bowl and add milk, oil, and honey. Beat well. Gradually beat in the dry ingredients. Pour into a nonstick 9×9-inch pan. Bake in a preheated 375° F oven for 25 minutes.

NUTRITION PER SERVING

		Calories:	143		
Carbohydrate:	21 g	Cholesterol:	23 mg	Potassium:	69 mg
Protein:	3 g	Fiber:	1.3 g	Calcium:	44 mg
Total Fat:	5 g	Sodium:	187 mg	Iron:	.7 mg

19

FAST AND FANCY NATURAL DESSERTS

ITALIANS NOT ONLY HAVE THE HEALTHIEST cuisine in the world, but also have the best idea of how to finish a family meal. They just pass a bowl of fresh fruit and nuts. We hope you will do the same most of the time or skip dessert altogether.

Sometimes it's not what you serve but how you serve it. When fresh berries are in season, place them in a stemmed wineglass and top with a dollop of yogurt and a sprinkling of nutmeg and grated lemon rind. Or cut up several kinds of melon and other fresh fruit and with a sprinkling of slivered almonds. Cut a grapefruit in half, scoop out the fruit and cut it up—add orange sections and some grapes and return all to be served in the grapefruit shell. Garnish with a sprig of mint.

However, there will be times when you would like to serve a cooked fruit, cookie, or cake and still want to conform to the Mood-Control Diet. This chapter is for those moments. You will find a sherbet without sugar or artificial sweetening, a dried fruit compote sweetened with honey, and some lower fat and no-white-sugar baked goods. Most of the recipes in chapter 18 could also be used as an occasional dessert. Freeze the extra portions of cookies, quick breads, and cake for another special treat.

TAKING A CLOSE LOOK AT DESSERTS

Here are calorie, fat, and sodium values for a serving of some popular desserts.* You will notice that serving sizes for different desserts are quite variable. For example, a serving of cheesecake is usually about half the size of a serving of apple pie.

Food	Calories	Fat (g)	Sodium (mg)
Fresh fruit cup	100	trace	trace
1/6 apple pie	405	18	475
3/4 cup chocolate mousse	280	21	55
1/12 cheesecake	280	18	205

Source: USDA Human Nutrition Information Service.

BAKED APPLES WITH RAISINS

(dairy-free, egg-free, gluten-free, sugar-free, yeast-free)   *Makes 4 servings*

Baked apples can be served hot or cold. Top with a dollop of yogurt, if desired, but not for dairy-free dieters.

INGREDIENTS
4 baking apples
4 teaspoons raisins
1/4 teaspoon cinnamon
1/2 cup water

Wash and core apples. Place in an 8×8-inch baking dish. Fill each apple cavity with a teaspoon of raisins and a dash of cinnamon. Pour water around apples. Bake in a 350° F oven for 35 minutes, or until fork tender.

NUTRITION PER SERVING
Calories: 134

Carbohydrate:	33 g	Cholesterol:	0 mg	Potassium:	255 mg
Protein:	trace	Fiber:	2 g	Calcium:	17 mg
Total Fat:	1 g	Sodium:	3 mg	Iron:	.7 mg

POACHED PEARS

(dairy-free, egg-free, gluten-free, sugar-free, yeast-free)   *Makes 4 servings*

If you would like the liquid to be thicker, remove the pears when they are finished cooking and simmer the liquid until reduced and thickened. This can be served hot or cold.

INGREDIENTS
4 pears
1 tablespoon white seedless raisins
1 cup water
1 teaspoon lemon juice
Dash of nutmeg
Dash of cinnamon

Cut pears in half. Remove peel and pits. Place in a large skillet with raisins, water, lemon juice, nutmeg, and cinnamon. Cover and cook over low heat until pears are tender, about 20 minutes.

NUTRITION PER SERVING

		Calories:	107		
Carbohydrate:	27 g	Cholesterol:	0 mg	Potassium:	231 mg
Protein:	1 g	Fiber:	2.3 g	Calcium:	14 mg
Total Fat:	1 g	Sodium:	3 mg	Iron:	.6 mg

BROILED HONEYED GRAPEFRUIT

(dairy-free, egg-free, gluten-free, yeast-free)   *Makes 2 servings*

When you have nothing but grapefruit halves, and you want to glamorize that a bit, think of broiling them with honey. Nutritious and delicious! Yeast-free dieters and hypoglycemics can broil the grapefruit without the honey.

INGREDIENTS
1 seedless grapefruit
2 teaspoons honey
1/2 teaspoon cinnamon

Cut grapefruit in half. Spread each cut top of grapefruit with 1 teaspoon of the honey. Sprinkle with cinnamon. Broil on broiler rack for 10 minutes, or until lightly browned. Serve at once.

NUTRITION PER SERVING

		Calories:	67		
Carbohydrate:	18 g	Cholesterol:	0 mg	Potassium:	162 mg
Protein:	1 g	Fiber:	.2 g	Calcium:	20 mg
Total Fat:	trace	Sodium:	1 mg	Iron:	.5 mg

BAKED AMBROSIA

(egg-free, gluten-free, sugar-free, yeast-free)   *Makes 4 servings*

Orange shells become the serving cup in this baked fruit appetizer. You can prepare this ahead of time and bake it just before serving.

INGREDIENTS
2 oranges
1/4 cup pitted cut-up dates
2 tablespoons coconut
1/4 cup chopped walnuts
1/2 cup plain nonfat yogurt
1/2 teaspoon vanilla extract

Cut oranges in half and scoop out the fruit, leaving the half shells intact. In a medium bowl mix orange segments with dates, coconut, and walnuts. Spoon fruit mixture back into the orange shells and place in an 8×8-inch baking dish. Bake in a 350° F oven for 25 minutes. Remove from oven. Stir yogurt and vanilla together in a small bowl, beating a little to make the mixture fluffy. Spoon some on top of each baked orange. Serve at once.

NUTRITION PER SERVING

		Calories:	136		
Carbohydrate:	20 g	Cholesterol:	.5 mg	Potassium:	316 mg
Protein:	4 g	Fiber:	.8 g	Calcium:	98 mg
Total Fat:	5 g	Sodium:	1 mg	Iron:	.9 mg

APPLESAUCE

(dairy-free, egg-free, gluten-free, sugar-free, yeast-free)   *Makes 6 servings*

You will probably not want to bother making your own applesauce, preferring to purchase an unsweetened commercial product. But you should know it's easy to do and should have the option of making your own.

INGREDIENTS
6 large apples, quartered, peeled, and cored
3/4 cup water
2 tablespoons lemon juice
1/4 teaspoon cinnamon, approximately

Place quartered apples in a medium-size, heavy saucepan with water, lemon juice, and cinnamon. Cover tightly and simmer over low heat until apples are mushy. Using a food mill, strain the sauce into a medium bowl. Add additional cinnamon to taste.

NUTRITION PER SERVING

		Calories:	126		
Carbohydrate:	31 g	Cholesterol:	0 mg	Potassium:	240 mg
Protein:	trace	Fiber:	2 g	Calcium:	15 mg
Total Fat:	1 g	Sodium:	2 mg	Iron:	.6 mg

HOT FRUIT COMPOTE

(dairy-free, egg-free, gluten-free, yeast-free)   *Makes 8 servings*

This hot fruit compote can be prepared ahead of time and reheated when needed. It is not necessary to flambé it, but it adds a bit of flair to do so! Sugar-free dieters should omit the honey and orange liqueur.

INGREDIENTS

1½ pounds mixed dried fruits, such as prunes, apricots, peaches, and pears
1½ cups cold water
1 tablespoon honey
2 tablespoons grated lemon rind
1 teaspoon cinnamon
¼ teaspoon nutmeg
3 tablespoons cornstarch
¼ cup orange liqueur

Cover dried fruits with the cold water in a medium bowl and let stand at room temperature for several hours or overnight. Drain off water from dried fruits into a medium-size saucepan or blazer pan of a chafing dish. Add honey, lemon rind, cinnamon, and nutmeg. Bring to a boil and cook for 10 minutes. Mix cornstarch and liqueur together until smooth; stir into mixture in pan. Add drained fruits; heat and stir until sauce is thickened. Serve fruit hot or cold, as a side dish to a main course or as a dessert.

To flambé, pour 1 ounce of brandy over fruit in a metal serving dish, and ignite with a match. Flame will flare up and then quickly die out. This is best done in the blazer of a chafing dish.

NUTRITION PER SERVING

		Calories:	140		
Carbohydrate:	32 g	Cholesterol:	0 mg	Potassium:	402 mg
Protein:	2 g	Fiber:	1 g	Calcium:	28 mg
Total Fat:	.2 g	Sodium:	10 mg	Iron:	2.2 mg

ORANGE-PINEAPPLE SHERBET

(egg-free, gluten-free, sugar-free, yeast-free)   *Makes 16 ¹/₂-cup servings*

If you'd like to cut down on sugar but do like a sweet ending to a meal, make your own sherbet. Here's a recipe that uses two kinds of frozen juice concentrate with no added sugar.

INGREDIENTS
1 (6-ounce) can frozen orange juice concentrate
1 (6-ounce) can frozen pineapple juice concentrate
3¹/₂ cups cold water
1 cup dry nonfat milk
1 teaspoon vanilla extract

Put all ingredients into a large bowl and beat just enough to blend thoroughly. Pour into ice cube trays. Freeze 1 to 2 hours until half-frozen. Remove to a large chilled mixing bowl; using an electric mixer, beat on low speed until mixture is softened, then beat on high speed 3 to 5 minutes until creamy but not liquid. Pour into freezer containers or ice cube trays. Freeze until ready to serve.

NUTRITION PER SERVING
Calories: 74

Carbohydrate:	17 g	Cholesterol:	0 mg	Potassium:	220 mg
Protein:	2 g	Fiber:	.08 g	Calcium:	54 mg
Total Fat:	.2 g	Sodium:	.8 mg	Iron:	.3 mg

SUNFLOWER-BRAN BALLS

(*dairy-free, egg-free, yeast-free*)   *Makes 18 cookies*

Here's a way to make cookies without having to bake them. The nice part is that they are made from highly nutritious ingredients. Because of the honey, this is not for sugar-free dieters.

INGREDIENTS
3 cups wheat bran flake cereal
1/4 cup toasted wheat germ
1/2 cup seedless raisins
2/3 cup creamy peanut butter
3 tablespoons orange juice
2 tablespoons honey
1/4 cup shelled sunflower seed

Crush bran flakes finely into a medium bowl. Add remaining ingredients and mix well. Shape into 18 balls and chill.

NUTRITION PER COOKIE
Calories: 112

Carbohydrate:	13 g	Cholesterol:	0 mg	Potassium:	152 mg
Protein:	4 g	Fiber:	.5 g	Calcium:	14 mg
Total Fat:	6 g	Sodium:	115 mg	Iron:	1.5 mg

CARROT COOKIES

(dairy-free, sugar-free, yeast-free)   *Makes 2 dozen cookies*

Save this for a day when your total fat intake is low. Just a sprinkling of cinnamon over the top of each cookie is all that's needed for this sugar-free snack.

INGREDIENTS
½ pound carrots, scraped and grated
1 cup corn oil margarine
3 eggs, lightly beaten
1 cup unbleached flour
2 teaspoons baking powder
½ teaspoon salt
½ cup ground walnuts
Cinnamon

Combine grated carrots with margarine in a large bowl; beat until fluffy. Add eggs and beat well. Sift flour, baking powder, and salt together; add to carrot mixture. Add ground walnuts and knead mixture on a floured board into a stiff dough. Divide dough in half and place each piece on a sheet of wax paper. Roll into a thick sausagelike roll, about 2 inches in diameter, using the wax paper as the outer wrapping. Unwrap and slice the dough into ¼-inch thick rounds. Place the rounds on nonstick cookie sheets, 1 inch apart. Lightly sprinkle tops with cinnamon. Bake in 350° F oven for 15 minutes, or until edges are lightly browned.

NUTRITION PER COOKIE

		Calories:	117		
Carbohydrate:	5 g	Cholesterol:	34 mg	Potassium:	59 mg
Protein:	3 g	Fiber:	.1 g	Calcium:	15 mg
Total Fat:	10 g	Sodium:	177 mg	Iron:	.5 mg

ORANGE CARROT CAKE

(dairy-free, yeast-free)   *Makes 16 servings*

Somehow if there are carrots in the cake, it sounds more nutritious. And it probably is! Don't bother with frosting—the cake has honey for sweetness (this recipe is not for hypoglycemics or the yeast sensitive).

INGREDIENTS

1 cup vegetable shortening
1/2 cup honey
1 teaspoon cinnamon
1/4 teaspoon nutmeg
1 tablespoon grated orange rind
4 eggs
1 1/2 cups grated scraped carrots
2/3 cup finely chopped walnuts
3 cups unbleached flour
1 tablespoon baking powder
1/2 teaspoon salt
1/3 cup orange juice

In a large bowl cream shortening and honey together until mixture is fluffy. Add cinnamon, nutmeg, and orange rind. Beat in eggs, one at a time. Add carrots and nuts. Sift flour, baking powder, and salt together. Add sifted flour mixture to the carrot mixture alternately with the orange juice, ending with flour. Mix well. Pour batter into lightly greased and floured 10-inch tube pan. Bake in a 350° F oven for 60 to 65 minutes, or until toothpick inserted in cake comes out clean. Cool in pan for 15 minutes, then turn out of pan and finish cooling on a wire rack.

NUTRITION PER SERVING

Calories: 288

Carbohydrate:	29 g	Cholesterol:	68 mg	Potassium:	113 mg
Protein:	6 g	Fiber:	.3 g	Calcium:	32 mg
Total Fat:	17 g	Sodium:	150 mg	Iron:	1.2 mg

20

SPECIAL PROBLEM AND FOOD-FIXER SECTION

THERE ARE MANY ILLNESSES THAT RE-spond directly to food manipulation or that will respond to other specific treatments better when the diet is optimal. In general, the week 3 menu plan of the Mood-Control Diet is optimal for maintaining health. When certain modifications are made in the diet, as noted in previous chapters, the week 3 diet plan becomes a therapeutic diet. In addition to alleviating depression and fatigue, there are many other medical conditions in which diet plays an important preventive or curative role.

This is not to imply that diet is all that is necessary to eradicate an illness. The following list is intended only to elevate the diet to its rightful place as a supportive or therapeutic tool in the treatment of illness and the maintenance of health. Please understand that the following list is not meant as a total treatment guide, for example, the use of special and general nutritional supplements is not discussed in the treatment of several illnesses.

The person in charge of your treatment should be your physician, but the overall results are usually improved when the patient is a knowledgable participant.

Special Problem	*Food Fixer*
Acne Vulgaris	Avoid fat and increase fiber, as in the week 3 menu plan.
Alcoholism	Causes depletion of nutrients and possible liver damage. Use hypoglycemic diet modifications of the week 3 menu plan. Seek counseling or group therapy.
Anorexia Nervosa	Psychological condition can lead to starvation habits causing malnutrition. The week 3 menu plan provides good nutrition, but counseling is also needed for best results.
Anxiety	Eliminate intake of alcohol, caffeine, and sugar. The week 3 menu plan should be helpful. Counseling may be necessary.

Arthritis	Avoid fat and possible trigger food(s) sensitivities. The week 3 menu plan should be helpful.
Atherosclerosis	Avoid saturated fat. Avoid margarines and shortenings. Decrease total fat intake to 20 to 30 percent of calories. The week 3 menu plan should be helpful.
Bulimia	This is a psychological problem manifested in food binges and self-induced purging. This condition can lead to malnutrition, and continual vomiting can destroy esophagus lining. Get counseling. Use week 3 menu plan to learn how to balance food intake.
Cancer	Increase fiber and beta-carotene (dark green and yellow fruits and vegetables) for possible prevention of large bowel cancer. Follow week 3 menu plan to provide better nutrition.
Cardiac Arrhythmias	Avoid caffeine. Have doctor check for possible cause from medication interaction.
Celiac Disease	*See Gluten Intolerance*.
Constipation	Increase dietary fiber. (See high fiber chart in appendix 3.)
Diabetes	Avoid sugar and fat. Increase dietary fiber. Eat four evenly spaced meals a day. Seek medical care.
Fibrocystic Breast Disease	Strictly avoid caffeine, including coffee, tea, chocolate, and cola drinks.
Food Sensitivity	See doctor and/or detect trigger food(s). Note 4-Day Rotation Diet on page 28. Avoid your trigger food(s).
Gallbladder Disease	Increase dietary fiber, avoid refined carbohydrates and excess fat.
Gluten Intolerance	Avoid wheat, rye, barley, and possibly oats. Use Grain Equivalency Table (page 247) for baking, if necessary.
Gout	Avoid red meat, organ meats, dried lentils, beans, and peas. Have medical tests for uric acid abnormality.
Heartburn	Avoid alcohol, chocolate, coffee, and fat.
Hiatal Hernia	Avoid heavy meals and spicy food. Many small meals are preferable to three large ones.

High Cholesterol	Limit cholesterol intake to 300 milligrams a day. Avoid saturated fat. Use polyunsaturated and monounsaturated fat instead. Eat more fish, less red meat. Limit egg yolks. Use the week 3 menu plan.
Hyperkinesis	Avoid sugar, food additives, and dyes. Test for trigger food(s) sensitivities.
Hypertension	Avoid sodium and saturated fat. Have adequate calcium intake. If taking prescribed diuretics include high-potassium food choices. Use the week 3 menu plan.
Insomnia	Avoid caffeine and alcohol.
Lactose Intolerance	See doctor about possible need for calcium supplementation. Avoid milk and dairy products. Follow the week 3 menu plan, using only dairy-free recipes.
Migraine Headaches	Avoid red wine and cheese because of tyramine content. Avoid monosodium glutamate (MSG) and excess sodium. Avoid caffeine.
Obesity	Reduce fat, sugar, and sodium intake. Eat less calories and increase exercise to rev up metabolism.
Premenstrual Syndrome	Reduce sodium intake. Avoid alcohol and caffeine.

These are but a few instances where a proper diet may contribute to the return or maintenance of health. The week 3 menu plan provides a healthy mixture of protein, fats, complex carbohydrates, and fiber. If you follow this plan, the usual offenders in your diet—sugar, caffeine, alcohol, and saturated fat—will be eliminated. The week 3 menu plan is a basic diet for good health.

SOURCES OF FURTHER INFORMATION

YEAST-FREE/SUGAR-FREE NUTRITIONAL SUPPLEMENTS

Klaire Laboratories, Inc. (Vital Life Co.)
1573 West Seminole
San Marcos, CA 92069
(619) 744–9680

Willner Chemists, Inc.
330 Lexington Ave.
New York, NY 10016
(212) 685–2538

CANDIDA TESTING INFORMATION

Immunodiagnostic Laboratories, Inc.
P.O. Box 5755
San Leandro, CA 94577
(415) 635–4555

ALLERGY TESTING INFORMATION

Immuno-Nutritional Clinical Laboratory
6700 Valjean Ave.
Van Nuys, CA 91406
(800) 344–4646 outside California
(800) 542–8855 within California

PHYSICIAN REFERRALS

(United States)   The Huxley Institute for Biosocial Research
900 North Federal Highway, Suite 330
Boca Raton, FL 33432
(407) 393–6167

(Canada)   Canadian Schizophrenia Foundation
7375 Kingsway
Burnaby, BC, Canada V3N 3B5
(604) 521–1728

271

SELECTED LIST OF RESOURCES:

United States Department of Agriculture
Human Nutrition Information Service
6505 Belcrest Road
Hyattsville, MD 20782

National Institutes of Health
National Cancer Institute
Bethesda, MD 20892

Canadian Bureau of Nutritional Sciences
Health and Welfare Canada
Brooke Claxton Building
Tunney's Pasture
Ottawa, K1A 0K9, Canada

Plant Fiber in Foods (1986), James W. Anderson, M.D.
Nutrition Research Foundation
Box 22124
Lexington, KY 40522

The Missing Diagnosis (1983), C. Orian Truss, M.D.
Missing Diagnosis, Inc.
PO Box 26508
Birmingham, AL 35226

The Allergic Gourmet (1983), June Roth, M.S.
Contemporary Books, Inc.
180 North Michigan Ave.
Chicago, IL 60601

Eat Right, Be Bright (1988)
Arthur Winter, M.D., and Ruth Winter
St. Martin's Press
175 Fifth Avenue
New York, NY 10010

The Food Sensitivity Diet (1984), Doug A. Kaufmann
Freundlich Books
80 Madison Ave.
New York, NY 10016

Coping With Your Allergies (1979),
Natalie Golos and Frances Golos Golbitz
Simon & Schuster
1230 Avenue of Americas
New York, NY 10020

Hypoglycemia: The Disease Your Doctor Won't Treat (1980)
Harvey M. Ross, M.D. and Jeraldine Saunders
Pinnacle/Viking Press
40 West 23 St.
New York, NY 10011

Harvard Medical School Health Letter
PO Box 10943
Des Moines, IA 50340
University of Missouri-Columbia School of Medicine
Columbia, MO 65201

The Way Up from Down (1987), Pricilla Slagle, M.D.
Random House
201 East 50th St.
New York, NY 10022

Nutritional Influences on Illness (1987),
Melvyn R. Werbach, M.D.
Keats Publishing Inc.
27 Pine St.
New Canaan, CT 06840

A Year in Nutritional Medicine (1986),
Edited by Jeffrey Bland, Ph.D.
Keats Publishing Inc.
27 Pine St.
New Canaan, CT 06840

Orthomolecular Medicine for Physicians (1989),
Abram Hoffer, M.D., Ph. D.
Keats Publishing Inc.
27 Pine St.
New Canaan, CT 06840

Quick Reference to Clinical Nutrition (1979),
Edited by Seymour L. Halpern, M.D.
J. S. Lippincott Company
East Washington Square
Philadelphia, PA 19105

The Complete Book of Vitamins (1984),
Rodale Press Inc.
33 East Minor St.
Emmaus, PA 18049

Alcoholics Anonymous
General Service Office
PO Box 10459, Grand Central Station
New York, NY 10063

FOOD FAMILIES (BIOLOGICAL RELATIONSHIPS)

Algae Family
  Agar agar
  Kelp
  Seaweed
Arrowroot Family
  Arrowroot (Maranta starch)
Arum Family
  Ceriman
  Dasheen arrowroot
  Taro arrowroot (poi)
Banana Family
  Arrowroot
  Banana
  Plantain
Beech Family
  Chestnuts
Birch Family
  Filbert
  Wintergreen (oil)
Borage Family
  Borage
  Comfrey
Brassica (cruciferous) Family
  Broccoli
  Brussels sprout
  Cabbage
  Cauliflower
  Horseradish

Kale
Kohlrabi
Radish
Rutabaga
Turnip
Watercress
Buckthorn Family
  Grape
    Brandy
    Raisin
    Wine
    Wine vinegar
  Muscadine
Buckwheat Family
  Buckwheat
  Rhubarb
  Sorrel
Caper Family
  Caper
Carica Family
  Papaya
Carrot Family
  Anise
  Caraway
  Carrot
  Celeriac
  Celery
  Chervil

Cumin
Dill
Fennel
Lovage
Parsley
Parsnip
Cashew Family
  Cashew
  Mango
  Pistachio
Catcus Family
  Prickly pear
Grass Family
  Bamboo shoots
  Barley
    Malt
    Maltose
  Cane sugar
    Molasses
    Raw sugar
  Corn
    Cornmeal
    Corn oil
    Cornstarch
    Corn sugar
    Corn syrup
    Hominy grits
    Popcorn
  Hops
  Millet
  Oats
  Rice
  Rye
  Sorghum grain
    Sorghum syrup
  Wheat
    Bran
    Bulgur
    Flour
      Gluten
      Graham
      Whole wheat

    Wheat germ
  Wild rice
Composite Family
  Chamomile
  Chicory
  Dandelion
  Endive
  Escarole
  Globe artichoke
  Jerusalem artichoke
  Lettuce
  Romaine
  Safflower oil
  Salsify
  Santolina
  Sunflower oil
  Tansy
  Tarragon
  Wormwood (absinthe)
  Vermouth
Crustacean Family
  Crab
  Crayfish
  Lobster
  Prawn
  Shrimp
Cyperaceae Family
  Water chestnuts
Dillenia Family
  Chinese gooseberry
Ebony Family
  American persimmon
  Japanese persimmon (kaki)
Farinosa Family
  Pineapple
Fish Families—Freshwater
  Bass Family
    White perch
    Yellow bass
  Catfish Family
    Catfish
  Croaker Family

Drum
Herring Family
  Shad
    Roe
Minnow Family
  Carp
  Chub
Perch Family
  Sauger
  Walleye
  Yellow perch
Pike Family
  Muskellunge
  Pickerel
  Pike
Salmon Family
  Salmon
  Trout
Smelt Family
  Smelt
Sturgeon Family
  Sturgeon
    Caviar
Sunfish Family
  Black bass
  Crapple
  Sunfish
Whitefish Family
  Whitefish
Fish Families—Saltwater
Anchovy Family
  Anchovy
Bluefish Family
  Bluefish
Codfish Family
  Cod (scrod)
  Cusk
  Haddock
  Hake
  Pollack
Croaker Family
  Croaker

Drum
Sea trout
Silver perch
Spot
Spotted sea trout
Dolphin Family
  Dolphin
Eel Family
  American eel
Flounder Family
  Dab
  Flounder
  Halibut
  Plaice
  Sole
  Turbot
Harvest Fish Family
  Butterfish
  Harvest fish
Herring Family
  Menhaden
  Pilchard (sardine)
  Sea herring
Jack Family
  Amberjack
  Pompano
  Yellow jack
Mackerel Family
  Albacore
  Bonito
  Mackerel
  Skipjack
  Tuna
Marlin Family
  Marlin
  Sailfish
Mullet Family
  Mullet
Porgy Family
  Porgy (scup)
Scorpionfish Family
  Ocean perch (rosefish)

Sea Bass Family
  Grouper
  Sea bass
Sea Catfish Family
  Ocean catfish
Silverside Family
  Silverside (whitebait)
Swordfish Family
  Swordfish
Tilefish Family
  Tilefish
Fungus Family
  Bakers' yeast
  Brewers' yeast
  Morel
  Mushroom
  Truffle
Ginger Family
  Cardamom
  Ginger
  Turmeric
Ginseng Family
  Ginseng (American and
    Chinese)
Goosefoot Family
  Beet
  Chard
  Spinach
  Sugar beet
  Swiss chard
Gourd Family
  Cantaloupe
  Casaba melon
  Choyote
  Chinese melon
  Crenshaw melon
  Cucumber
  Honeydew melon
  Persian melon
  Pumpkin
  Squash
    Acorn

    Buttercup
    Butternut
    Crookneck
    Cushaw
    Hubbard
    Pattypan
    Turban
    Vegetable spaghetti
    Zucchini
  Watermelon
Heath Family
  Blueberry
  Cranberry
  Gooseberry
  Huckleberry
Honeysuckle Family
  Cranberry
  Elderberry
Iris Family
  Saffron (crocus)
Laurel Family
  Avocado
  Bay leaf
  Cinnamon
  Sassafras
Legume Family
  Alfalfa
  Beans
    Kidney
    Lima
    Mung
    Pinto
    Soybean
      Lecithin
      Soy flour
      Soy grits
      Soy milk
      Soy oil
  String
  Black-eyed pea
  Carob
  Chick-pea (garbanzo)

Lentil
Licorice
Pea
Peanut
Split pea
Lily Family
  Asparagus
  Chives
  Garlic
  Leek
  Onion
  Sarsaparilla
  Shallot
Madder Family
  Coffee
Mallow Family
  Cottonseed oil
  Okra
Mammal Families
  Bear Family
    Bear
  Bovine Family
    Beef
      Gelatin
      Oleomargarine
      Rennet
      Sausage casings
      Suet
      Calf (veal)
      Milk products
        Butter
        Cheese
        Cream
        Dried milk
        Ice Cream
        Milk (low-fat, skim, whole)
        Yogurt
    Buffalo
    Goat
      Cheese
      Milk
    Sheep

    Lamb
    Mutton
  Deer Family
    Caribou
    Deer (venison)
    Elk
    Moose
    Reindeer
  Hare Family
    Rabbit
  Horse Family
    Horse
  Opossum Family
    Opossum
  Pronghorn Family
    Antelope
  Squirrel Family
    Squirrel
  Swine Family
    Hog (pork)
    Bacon
    Ham
    Lard
    Pork gelatin
    Sausage
    Scrapple
  Whale Family
    Whale
Maple Family
  Maple sugar
Mint Family
  Apple mint
  Basil
  Catnip
  Horehound
  Lemon balm
  Marjoram
  Oregano
  Peppermint
  Rosemary
  Sage
  Spearmint

Summer Savory
Thyme
Winter Savory
Mollusk Family
  Abalone
  Clam
  Mussel
  Oyster
  Scallop
  Snail
  Squid
Morning Glory Family
  Sweet potato
Mulberry Family
  Breadfruit
  Fig
  Mulberry
Mustard Family
  Collard greens
  Mustard greens
    Mustard seed
Myristicaceae Family
  Nutmeg
  Mace
Myrtle Family
  Allspice
  Clove
  Eucalyptus
  Guava
Nightshade Family
  Bell pepper
  Cayenne pepper
  Chili pepper
  Eggplant
  Paprika
  Pimiento
  Potato (white)
  Tobacco
  Tomato
Olive Family
  Olive (green or ripe)
  Olive oil

Orchid Family
  Vanilla bean
Palm Family
  Coconut
    Coconut oil
  Date
  Palm Cabbage
Parsley Family
  Watercress
Passionflower Family
  Passion fruit
Pedalium Family
  Sesame seed
    Sesame oil
    Tahini
Pepper Family
  Black pepper
  White pepper
Pomegranate Family
  Pomegranate
    Grenadine
Poultry Family
  Chicken
    Eggs
  Duck
  Goose
  Pheasant
  Rock Cornish hen
  Turkey
Rose Family
  Almond
  Apple
  Apricot
  Blackberry
  Boysenberry
  Cherry
  Crabapple
  Dewberry
  Loganberry
  Nectarine
  Peach
  Pear

Plum
Prune
Quince
Raspberry
Rosehips
Strawberry
Rue Family
  Citron
  Grapefruit
  Kumquat
  Lemon
  Murcot
  Lime
  Orange
  Tangelo
  Tangerine
Sapodilla Family
  Chickle (gum)
Sapucaia Family
  Brazil nut
Saxifrage Family
  Currant
  Gooseberry
Soapberry Family

  Litchi nut
Spurge Family
  Cassava
  Castor bean
  Curry
  Tapioca
  Yucca
Sterculia Family
  Cocoa
  Chocolate
  Cola nut
Tea Family
  Black tea
Walnut Family
  Black walnut
  Butternut
  English walnut
  Heartnut
  Hickory nut
  Pecan
  Walnut
Verbena Family
  Lemon verbena

HIGH-FIBER FOOD LIST

High Fiber Foods	Serving Size	Fiber (g)
VEGETABLES		
Asparagus	½ cup	3.5
Avocado	½	2.2
Beans, baked	½ cup	11.0
Beans, kidney	½ cup	9.7
Beans, lima	½ cup	8.3
Beans, navy	½ cup	8.4
Beans, pinto	½ cup	8.9
Bean sprouts	½ cup	1.5
Beans, string	½ cup	2.1
Beets	½ cup	2.1
Broccoli	½ cup	3.2
Brussels sprouts	½ cup	2.3
Cabbage	½ cup	2.1
Carrots, raw	½ cup	1.8
Cauliflower	½ cup	1.6
Celery, raw	½ cup	1.1
Corn, canned	½ cup	6.0
Corn	Medium ear	5.2
Eggplant	½ cup	2.5
Kale	½ cup	1.3
Lentils	½ cup	2.0
Lettuce	6 leaves	0.7
Mushrooms	½ cup	0.9
Onions	½ cup	1.2
Parsnips	½ cup	3.0
Peas, black-eye	½ cup	12.0

Peas, green	½ cup	4.2
Potatoes, sweet	1 medium	6.0
Potatoes, white	1 medium	4.0
Radishes	½ cup	1.3
Spinach	½ cup	5.7
Squash, acorn	½ cup	4.0
Squash, zucchini	½ cup	2.0
Tomato, raw	1 medium	2.0
Turnip	½ cup	2.0

FRUIT

Apple	1 large	4.0
Applesauce	½ cup	2.6
Apricots	1 medium	0.8
Banana	1 medium	2.0
Blackberries	½ cup	5.0
Cantaloupe	¼ medium	1.6
Cherries	10	1.1
Dates, dried	5	3.1
Fig, dried	1 medium	2.4
Grapes, seedless	12	0.3
Grapefruit	½	0.8
Orange	1	1.6
Peach	1	2.3
Pear	1	5.0
Pineapple	½ cup	0.8
Plum	1	0.6
Prunes, dried	2	2.0
Raisins	¼ cup	2.4
Raspberries	½ cup	4.6
Strawberries	½ cup	1.5

GRAINS

Bread, cracked wheat	1 slice	2.1
Bread, French	1 slice	0.7
Bread, pumpernickel	1 slice	1.2
Bread, rye	1 slice	1.2
Bread, white	1 slice	0.7
Bread, whole wheat	1 slice	2.1
Cereal, bran, 40%	½ cup	3.5
Cereal, bran, 100%	⅓ cup	8.4
Cereal, cornflakes	½ cup	0.9

Cereal, oat bran	⅓ cup	4.0
Cereal, oatmeal	½ cup	2.0
Cereal, raisin bran	½ cup	3.0
Cereal, shredded wheat	1 biscuit	3.0
Crackers, graham	1 square	0.7
Popcorn	1 cup	1.0
Rice, brown	½ cup	2.4
Rice, white	½ cup	0.7

NUTS

Peanuts	¼ cup	2.9
Peanut butter	1 tablespoon	1.2
Walnuts	¼ cup	1.6

EGGS	0.0
FATS	0.0
FISH, POULTRY, MEAT	0.0

Source: Compiled from USDA Human Nutrition Information Services and other sources (see Selected List of Resources, Appendix 1).

QUICK GUIDE TO SODIUM IN FOODS

QUICK GUIDE TO READING LABELS FOR HIDDEN SODIUM

Sodium Chloride. Salt used in cooking and food processing

Monosodium Glutamate. MSG, used in cooking and food processing

Baking Powder. Used in breads and cakes

Baking Soda. Sodium bicarbonate or bicarbonate of soda, used in breads, cakes, sometimes added to vegetables to retain color, and also found in alkalizers

Brine. Salt and water solution used in food processing, canning, freezing, and pickling

Disodium Phosphate. Used in quick-cooking cereals and processed cheese

Sodium Alginate. Used in chocolate milk and ice cream for smooth texture

Sodium Benzoate. Used as a preservative in condiments

Sodium Hydroxide. Used in processing some fruits and vegetables, hominy, and ripe olives

Sodium Propionate. Used in pasteurized cheese and some breads and cakes

Sodium Sulfite. Used as a bleach for some fresh fruits, as a preservative for some dried fruits

LIST OF HIGH-SODIUM FOODS

Anchovies	Canned soups
Bacon	Catsup
Beef, chipped	Caviar
Beef, corned	Celery salt
Bouillon cubes	Cheese

Chili sauce
Cod, dried
Fish, salted and smoked
Frankfurters
Frozen dinners
Frozen vegetables, sauced
Garlic salt
Herring
Luncheon meats
Meat extracts
Meat, salted and smoked
Meat sauces
Meat tenderizers
Mustard, prepared

Nuts, salted
Olives
Onion salt
Pickles
Popcorn, salted
Potato chips
Pretzels
Salt
Salt pork
Sardines
Sauerkraut
Sausages
Soy sauce
Worcestershire sauce

LIST OF MODERATELY HIGH-SODIUM FOODS

Baking powder
Baking soda
Beets, beet greens
Beverage mixes
Bread, rolls, crackers
Butter, salted
Carrots
Celery
Clams
Crabs
Dandelion greens
Fish, canned
Kidneys
Lobster

Margarine, salted
Meat, canned
Molasses
Mustard greens
Oysters
Salad dressings
Scallops
Shrimp
Spinach
Swiss chard
Vegetables, canned
Vegetable juices
Waffles

RECIPE INDEX

INDEX